Tess Daly

4 Steps

to a happier, healthier you

EAT · BREATHE
MOVE · SLEEP

bantam

For anyone who
needs to take
a moment for
themselves.

xx

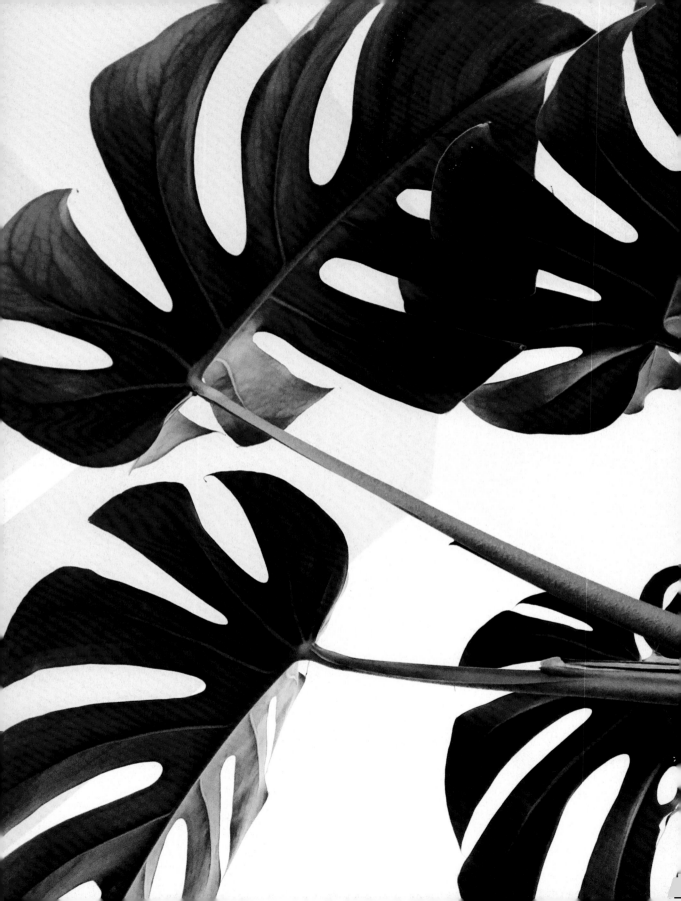

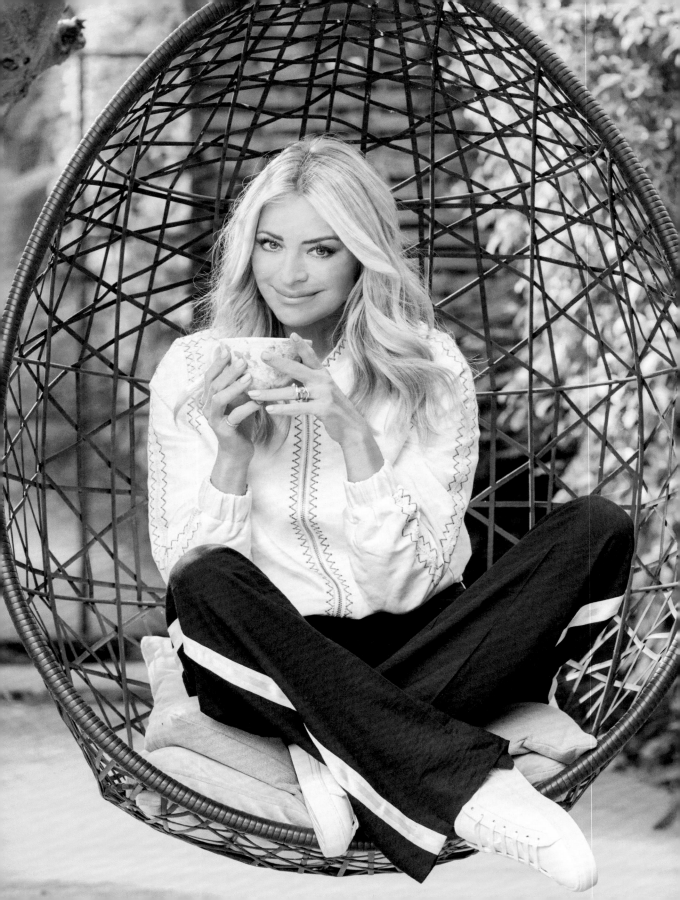

introduction

Do you ever find yourself thinking that life is just *so* busy? I know I do. From the moment we get up, we rush around, work our socks off – whether that's at home or in the office – dash from one thing to the next, and then we crash into bed. We lie awake worrying about what we have and haven't done. And then the cycle starts again when the morning alarm goes off. For so many of us, there never seems to be time for our own needs to come first.

Life is hectic and it can be hard to carve out moments of calm, to think about how *you're* feeling and take measures to create a little more 'me time'. It can seem like we're all running on empty and need the extra energy that comes with better health and feeling physically stronger. To this end, I believe that focusing on your wellbeing should be an absolute priority. With this book, I want to encourage everyone to do the seemingly little things that collectively make a *big* difference to our health and wellbeing.

We tend to think we don't have time to look after ourselves. There's always something else to do; something that feels more urgent, more important. If you're the main carer, you're the lynchpin for your family. Perhaps you don't have children, but your work or other obligations, such as caring for relatives, can take priority over looking after your own health. But if we're not at our best, it's harder to keep all those plates spinning.

Whatever your situation, this is your time to think about your own wellness. And if you can't do it for yourself, do it for everyone you love. If *you're* at your best, it helps everyone around you. We're all living longer, so let's try to live better too.

So, if you're feeling strung out or perhaps fed up with yo-yo-ing from one diet to the next, promising yourself that 'Next week I will move more, eat better and work less,' but you never quite get started, then I hope this is the book for you.

we're all living longer, so let's try to live better too

WELLBEING IS MY PASSION

I'm often asked, 'What do you do to look after yourself?' Perhaps this is due to the fact that despite reaching my fifties, I still find myself dashing around shiny studio floors in high heels and sparkly dresses. But after so many years of being judged on my appearance and seeing others judged the same way, I realized that the secret to feeling good was actually quite simple – it was what was happening *inside* my body that made me feel my absolute best.

true beauty is a healthy, happy body and mind

I'm convinced that wellness begins with nurturing ourselves from the inside out. I've come to the conclusion that true beauty comes from within: it's a healthy, happy body and mind and a kind heart. Let's nurture those lovely souls of ours with gratitude, good thoughts and a positive attitude and be rewarded with the feeling of a glorious lightness of being. Let's take time to breathe, to be in the moment – after all that is where the joy is; otherwise we're always seeking it outside ourselves. The route to good health is inside us, and I want to share the simple steps that have worked well for me.

To be our best selves, we need to look at four areas of our daily lives and what we can do for our mind and body through eating, breathing, moving and sleeping. Clearly, while I have a keen interest in health and have developed my own strategies, I'm not an expert. To gain more knowledge to share with you, I've consulted a professional in each field, and I'm grateful to have learnt so much about simple ways to improve my own wellbeing along the way.

EAT

I'm absolutely *fascinated* by the fact that the food we eat has the power to make us healthy. Food is the fuel that supercharges our bodies, and by thinking more about what we eat, we can reduce our risk of dietary-induced diseases. We really can eat ourselves well!

As the mother of girls, I've always been wary of using the word 'diet'. I believe in having a positive relationship with food, focusing on eating whole foods with plenty of fruit and veg. I encourage my daughters to eat healthy balanced meals and avoid calorie counting at all costs. I believe that moderation is key, and a little bit of what you fancy really won't hurt.

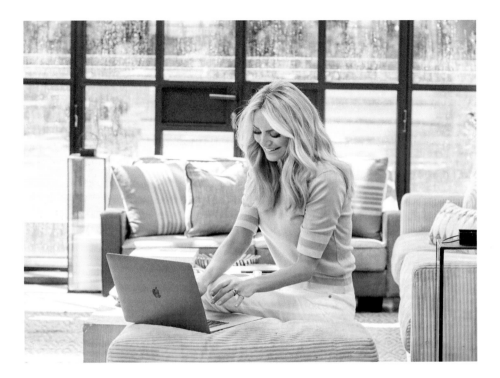

I've become particularly interested in gut health, a field of research that is proving to have huge implications for everything from our state of mind to our immune systems. Did you know that 70 per cent of your immune system is in your gut? To learn more, I spoke to leading nutritionist Dr Linia Patel, an expert on gut health. She has shared lots of information on questions such as how to eat for a healthy gut, the importance of fibre, how to reduce inflammation in the body and what really does make for a healthy diet.

I've also included a selection of recipes that I love to cook for my family. They're simple, delicious, nutritious and gut-friendly too.

BREATHE

Focusing on the way I breathe has opened up a whole new way of thinking about how my mind is connected to my body and how crucial such a simple but important wellbeing tool breathing can be. Deep breathing is vital for getting energy *into* and stress *out* of the body. Stress is damaging to us – it makes us feel tired and lacking in energy, and it can lead to serious illness. It can affect the immune system too, so the less stressed we are, the healthier it makes us.

For help, I consulted breathwork coach Rebecca Dennis, who immediately told me I was a shallow breather and explained how I could help myself with breathing exercises. She has shared her expertise and provided lots of simple techniques to help us all reduce stress and improve our wellbeing.

MOVE

Staying active is an all-important game-changer for good health and I don't necessarily mean hitting the gym, although that's great if it works for you. I'm talking about those simple life hacks that get us moving just that bit more than yesterday. Things we can do at home, without special clothes or equipment. You don't have to be an Olympic athlete – something as simple as a daily walk and some stretches can make a big difference.

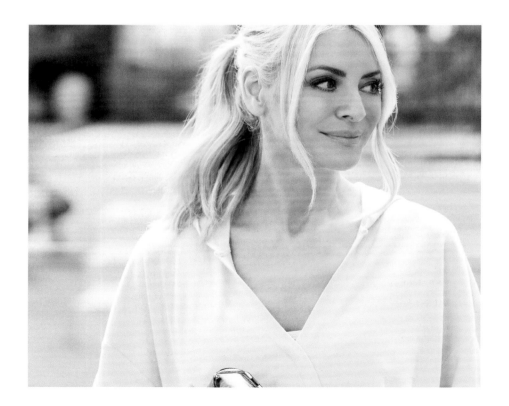

And get this for a wake-up call! Experts now say that *sitting* is the new *smoking* and so even just standing up while you're on the phone or balancing on one leg while you wait for the kettle to boil can genuinely help. I used to think I was too busy to exercise, but now I know better, and I've shared the tips and hacks that have worked for me, plus some advice on home routines from Sam Shaw, an expert personal trainer. Give them a try and you'll soon feel the benefit.

SLEEP

I used to skimp on sleep – I didn't understand its importance and viewed it as an inconvenience, something that got in the way. Then I became a parent – a sleep-deprived new parent! – and for the first time, I discovered just what real tiredness felt like and the relevance of sleep to maintaining good health. Through sheer necessity, I began to take it more seriously and developed strategies for getting a better night's rest.

Dr Linia Patel began to study sleep when she realized that some of her clients, despite having a good diet and plenty of exercise, weren't reaching optimal health because they weren't sleeping enough. She has helped me to understand much more about why we sleep and how modern life and stress can disrupt our normal sleep cycles.

SMALL STEPS – BIG CHANGES

In researching and writing this book, I've realized just how important it is for us all to feel good about ourselves in order to get the most out of life. I want to help you make great choices that fit in with your lifestyle. My plan is simple and straightforward, with lots of practical tips and tricks that have worked for me, and I hope can work for you too. There's nothing complicated or difficult about it. Wellbeing can be an everyday part of our busy lives. Don't feel you have to change everything overnight. Start small and build up gradually, so that eating better, moving more and giving extra thought to your breathing and sleep quality become a routine part of your life. Small steps can add up to big changes. I hope they empower and inspire you to live the happiest and healthiest life you can.

my plan is simple and straightforward

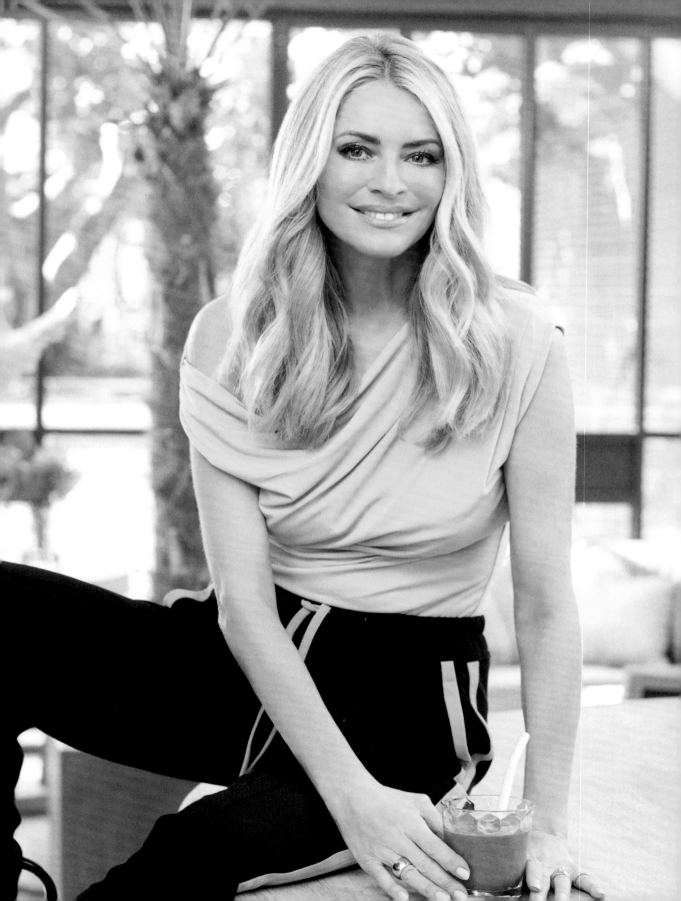

EAT

**Getting your nutrition
right is a journey**

the healing properties of food

I started my working life as a model in the fashion industry, a world not known for its good relationship with food. For me, though, dieting was never an option. I saw too many friends sabotage their health through crash diets for a quick fix or because some agent had carelessly said, 'You need to lose a bit of weight.' Worse still, I saw others suffer from anorexia. I understood that fad diets of any kind were not the way to happiness and were actually pretty detrimental to your health. I've never dieted. I feel many diets are unrealistic to maintain and only lead to misery, and that's why I refuse to include calorie information for the recipes in this book.

I've always loved my food, but I didn't realize quite what a difference eating well could make to my health and my body. I was first introduced to the healing properties of food years ago through an amazing book I found in a flea market when living in New York. It was called *The Food Pharmacy* and it contained information about the healthful properties of foods and wonderfully colourful recipes with medicinal properties.

I've always loved my food

The first recipe I tried was an 'immune-boosting bruschetta' – toasted rye bread drizzled with extra virgin olive oil and rubbed with a raw garlic clove, then topped with chopped cherry tomatoes, avocado and fresh basil leaves. It tasted like a little piece of heaven and it was a revelation that I could supercharge my immunity by eating something so absolutely utterly delicious. Good food, healthy food, didn't have to be bland or boring.

At that time, I was living in one of the world's most polluted cities, so the idea that I could boost my immune system while enjoying my food was a real win-win. What's more, harmful food additives and colourings that had long been banned in the UK and Europe were still being used in the USA then, and avoiding them was like playing Russian roulette. Obesity and disease were constantly being discussed on the news and I was determined to seek out healthy options when it came to the foods I ate, and that book really helped get me on the right path.

CARING FOR OURSELVES MEANS CARING FOR OUR GUT

It's only in the last decade that scientific research has shown that our gut rules our health. A healthy gut means a healthy body. What's more, good food equals good mood because the gut – sometimes referred to as our second brain – also governs our thoughts, feelings and emotions, due to the hormones it produces. What we eat affects who we are, and we are discovering that caring for ourselves means caring for our gut.

I want my daughters to grow up strong and confident, not worrying about how they look, and I try to teach them that health starts from the inside. It may not sound very glamorous, but nurturing your gut is what will bring you glowing skin and glossy hair on the outside as well as a strong immune system on the inside. Our gut affects everything about our body, from the way we feel to our ability to stay healthy. A healthy body is a beautiful body and good gut health shows itself in every aspect of your being.

Ever since that first heavenly bruschetta, I've become passionately interested in gut health. To find out more I spoke with Dr Linia Patel, an eminent dietitian who has a wide range of clients, including athletes, business tycoons and NHS workers. She told me that when she was training, the whole issue of our gut health wasn't even mentioned. Incredibly, it only started being talked about seven or eight years ago. Before then, the gut was seen just as a tube that our food passed through and where it got digested, absorbed and excreted.

a healthy
body is a
beautiful
body

GET TO KNOW YOUR GUT

We all know roughly how the digestive system works, but maybe it's worth clarifying before talking more about the gut:

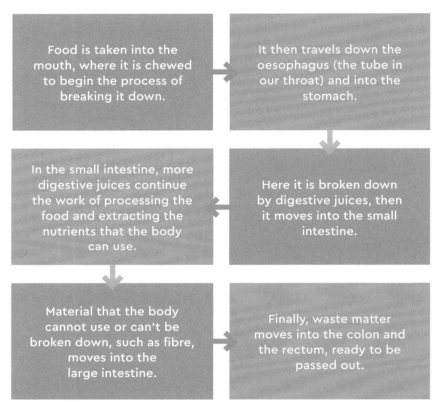

Food is taken into the mouth, where it is chewed to begin the process of breaking it down.

It then travels down the oesophagus (the tube in our throat) and into the stomach.

In the small intestine, more digestive juices continue the work of processing the food and extracting the nutrients that the body can use.

Here it is broken down by digestive juices, then it moves into the small intestine.

Material that the body cannot use or can't be broken down, such as fibre, moves into the large intestine.

Finally, waste matter moves into the colon and the rectum, ready to be passed out.

Research has shown that people who eat a good, balanced diet, a diet that's rich in plant-based foods, are less likely to die of heart problems and cancer. And recent research even shows that Alzheimer's could be linked to what you eat. Good gut health is also essential for our resistance to disease. Linia shared with me the incredible fact that we now know that there are more bacterial cells in our body than human cells. These microbes in your gut not only help your body digest food but also help regulate your metabolism and your immune system. In fact, almost 70 per cent of your immune system is in your gut. These good bacteria influence your body's T-cells, the crucial white blood cells that help power your immune system. They also help reduce inflammation, which prevents infection.

70 per cent of your immune system is in your gut

GOOD GUT
HEALTH IS
ESSENTIAL FOR
OUR RESISTANCE
TO DISEASE.

the story of the gut

I've long been fascinated by the diets of different people around the globe, by those who seem to live longer, healthier lives than average, such as people in the so-called blue zones. These are regions of the world where many more people than usual live to over 100 and include areas of Japan, Sardinia, Costa Rica and Greece. Common characteristics of the lifestyles in these regions are staying active, eating lots of fruit and vegetables, and not overeating.

Linia told me that at the beginning of the research into the gut, scientists began to notice the connection between mental health, inflammation and the Standard American Diet (SAD), which is made up of very refined, ultra-processed foods, low in fibre and high in saturated fat and added sugar. This diet seems to cause inflammation and is linked with lower scores in mood and memory, and higher rates of depression. They compared this with a traditional sub-Saharan diet, looking at hunter-gatherers in Tanzania living a very simple life. These people are outdoors a lot, eat plenty of fibre and plant food, and were found to have higher scores in mental wellbeing, and lower levels of inflammation, than the American sample.

THREE DAYS TO CHANGE YOUR GUT BACTERIA

The scientists then conducted an experiment – switching a group of American volunteers to a Tanzanian diet and vice versa. After three days, they started seeing changes and these changes were linked to gut microbiota – the bacteria in the gut. Incredibly, it takes just three days to change the gut bacteria for better or worse. It seems that we don't run ourselves, our gut bacteria run us. The old adage was 'You are what you eat.' The truth is that you are what your gut bacteria eat and thrive on.

You might have thought of all bacteria as harmful, but they are not. They are vital to our bodies and there are trillions of them all over the skin and in the body, but particularly in our gut, where they are referred to as our gut flora.

'There are roughly 40 trillion bacterial cells in your body and only 30 trillion human cells,' Linia told me. 'This means that we are more bacteria than human. Most of these bacteria live in a pocket of the large intestine called the caecum and they are referred to as the gut microbiome. Your microbiome plays an important role in your wellbeing, your health and the strength of your immune system and each person's gut microbiome is unique.'

But it is not just our food that affects our gut bacteria. Stress levels, sleep quality, antibiotic use, whether you have pets or not, even how you were born (vaginal or C-section birth) and many other factors have an impact on the balance of good and bad bacteria in the gut.

Baby-feeding methods also make a difference and breastfeeding seems to foster the growth of diverse gut bacteria. And children whose parents are fanatical about cleanliness and use antibacterial sprays may have a less diverse gut bacteria than those who are allowed to play outside and get dirty.

the truth is you are what your gut bacteria eat

Gut bacteria thrive on:

+ a good variety of plant-based foods

+ fibre

+ wholegrains

+ phytonutrients in fruit and vegetables

They don't thrive on:

+ lots of added sugar or refined carbohydrates

+ lots of saturated fat

+ alcohol

+ habitual intake of artificial sweeteners

+ lots of ultra-processed foods

Linia stresses that by recommending a plant-based diet for gut health, she is not saying necessarily to go vegetarian or vegan – just to include plenty of fruit and veg, pulses and nuts, and small amounts of meat and dairy, if you wish. It's all about moderation. Eat healthily most of the time, then if you want a crumpet or a chocolate bar in the afternoon, that's fine, as long as it doesn't become an everyday habit. Don't deprive yourself but listen to your gut and think about what's best.

That's always been my approach. I've never dieted but my mum's nickname for me was 'I'll have half' because when I was in my later teenage years, that's what I would do. There was always half a chocolate orange or half a chocolate bar in the fridge. That was my way of letting myself have what I wanted, without overdoing it. I've always believed the saying 'A little of what you fancy does you good.' For me, moderation is key.

FIBRE

All important for gut health is fibre. It helps to increase our gut bacteria and a diet high in fibre seems to reduce inflammation in the body and reduce the risk of illnesses such as heart disease and diabetes. Linia explained that fibre is basically a part of any plant-based food that remains undigested in our gut and then gets excreted. There are two main types of fibre – soluble and insoluble. You need some of both types for a healthy gut, plus some of what are termed prebiotic fibre foods, which are particularly beneficial for gut bacteria.

Soluble fibre

As the name suggests, soluble fibre dissolves in water and forms a gel-like substance in the gut. This helps to slow down digestion and keeps us feeling fuller for longer.

Good sources of soluble fibre include:

+ oats
+ bananas
+ strawberries
+ mushrooms
+ peas

+ beans
+ apples
+ citrus fruit
+ carrots
+ barley

Insoluble fibre

Insoluble fibre does not dissolve. It passes through the digestive system and bulks up your stools, while keeping them soft so they can be passed more easily.

Good sources of insoluble fibre include:

+ wholewheat flour
+ wheat bran
+ nuts
+ beans

+ cauliflower
+ green beans
+ potatoes with skins on
+ apples and pears with skins on

Many foods, of course, contain both types of fibre. Apples are a good example. The apple skin contains insoluble fibre and the inside is soluble fibre. Plenty of fibre also helps us balance blood glucose levels and manage cholesterol, reducing bad or LDL cholesterol. The official recommendation is that for good gut health, adults should have about 30g of fibre a day, but too many of us are not managing that.

Be careful, though. If you suffer from bowel or digestive problems, check with your doctor or a qualified dietitian before increasing your fibre intake.

how to add fibre to your diet

Breakfast

- **Start with whole oats**. A medium bowl of porridge topped with a handful of berries gives you 8g of fibre. Boost your fibre further by adding a tablespoon of chia or ground flaxseed (4g fibre).

- **Make a vegetable omelette**. Try to add two portions of vegetables (2 × 80g/2¾oz) to your omelette and this will give you about 8g of fibre. Use whatever vegetables you have – fresh, frozen or tinned.

Lunch

- **Lean on lentils or beans and veggies.** Try having lentils or beans instead of rice or pasta (120g/4¼oz of legumes gives you 10g fibre). Or if you're not a lentils or beans fan, why not add some veggies to the rice or pasta while it boils (add 80g/2¾oz veggies to get 3–4g fibre).

- **Choose wholegrain**. Where possible, opt for wholegrain varieties as they will have a higher amount of fibre per serving. Think wholegrain bread, pasta, brown or red rice, wholegrain couscous, quinoa or oatcakes. If you have potatoes, keep the skins on.

Evening meal

- **Base your meal on veggies**. A 250g (9oz) mixed vegetable stir-fry with 120g (4¼oz) chicken will give you 10g of fibre.

- **Have soupy suppers**. Cook up a vegetable soup using any leftover vegetables you have. This includes fresh, frozen or tinned. One serving (250ml/9fl oz) of mixed vegetable soup can give you up to 5g fibre.

Snacks

- **Snack on fibre**. What raw vegetables do you have in your fridge that you can snack on? 150g (5½oz) of sugar snap peas or raw carrots provide you with 4g of fibre. 150g (5½oz) raspberries provide 10g fibre. A medium apple and 30g (1oz) unsalted nuts provide 6g of fibre.

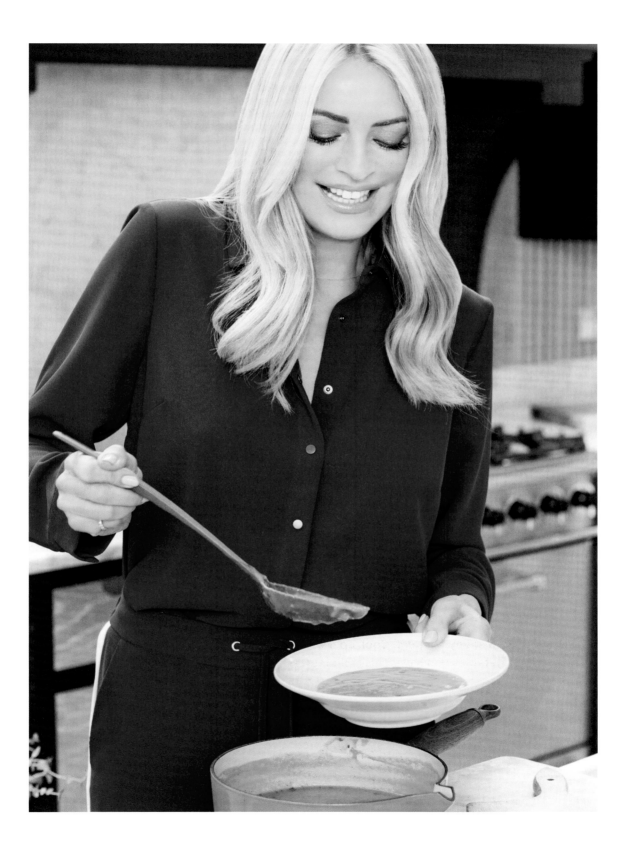

When it comes to increasing the amount of fibre in your diet, there are some things worth bearing in mind:

- **Increase your intake slowly and gradually.** It takes our large intestine time to adjust and adapt to an increased load of fibre. If you go too quickly, you may end up feeling super bloated and gassy. Increase your intake by one portion per day. After one week, add another and continue until you have reached your target.

- **Drink water.** Fibre needs water to work. So, if you are increasing your fibre intake, make sure you drink enough water too.

PREBIOTICS AND PROBIOTICS

Prebiotics
These are a particular kind of fibre that we cannot digest but which feed healthy bacteria in the gut. They have many benefits, including improving blood sugar balance, strengthening immunity and reducing inflammation in the body.

Examples of some prebiotic foods include:

+ Jerusalem artichokes
+ garlic
+ onions
+ leeks

+ asparagus
+ oats
+ barley
+ chicory root

Probiotics
These are foods that contain certain types of live bacteria to increase your gut flora.

Examples of probiotic foods include:

+ live yoghurt
+ kefir

+ fermented foods such as kimchi

SUPPLEMENTS

Generally speaking, Linia says that if you are aiming to manage something like a gut symptom it may be advisable to take a probiotic supplement, but it's best to talk to a registered dietitian or nutritionist to establish what would work best for you.

As to prebiotic supplements, Linia doesn't advise these for most people. She says the research tells us that having the naturally occurring prebiotics in food is the best way forward. There are some scenarios where a prebiotic supplement is recommended, but these are infrequent and should be taken on a case-by-case basis.

OUR GUT LOVES VARIETY

The 'five-a-day' message is great but it's important to have variety as well. Don't always go for the same vegetable and the same fruit. Mix it up as much as possible and choose different items to put in your shopping basket. One thing that helps is eating seasonally.

I know we've all become so used to the idea that we can have anything we want at any time of year, but when you think about it, what's the point of flying produce thousands of miles across the globe? Do we really need parsnips in August or strawberries in December? It's so much better to eat what's grown locally when it's in season. That way the food is fresher, tastes better and you help farmers and the planet – it's a win–win. My nearest town has a farmers' market every week and I take real pleasure in buying locally grown fruit and vegetables when they're in season and often much cheaper than supermarket prices.

Of course, there are some things that we can't grow here in the UK, like oranges and bananas, but as far as possible I try to cook and eat with the seasons and shop in markets and small stores where they sell locally grown produce. Eating seasonally also adds variety and interest to our meals – and we look forward to the first asparagus in April or May, beautiful berries in summer and lovely crisp apples in September.

30 PLANT POINTS A WEEK

American researchers found that people who eat about 30 different plant-based foods a week have a more diverse gut biome than those who are eating half that. 'I'm not claiming that 30 is a magic number,' Linia says, 'but the more different plant-based foods you eat over the week, the better for your health.' The idea works on a points system. Every time you eat a different 80g (2¾oz) portion of fruit or vegetable within the week counts as one point. Herbs and spices count for a quarter of a point each. Getting up to 30 points a week may sound daunting, but it needn't be. Here are some ideas:

- Use a range of different leaves in your green salads, instead of just lettuce. Try rocket, watercress, lamb's lettuce, baby spinach.

- Sneak extra veg into your cooking. Stir a handful of frozen peas or broad beans into a tomato sauce. Add some sweetcorn to a soup.

- Add some fresh herbs to your dishes – and don't just use parsley. Try coriander, dill, chives, basil and thyme.

- Sprinkle in some spice – turmeric is a great anti-inflammatory, for instance. To really get the benefits, you would need to take loads, but just adding a little to your daily diet is a move in the right direction. Ginger is another good anti-inflammatory. Try making a herbal tea by infusing some slices of fresh root ginger and lemon.

- Add some seeds to your food. Sunflower seeds and pumpkin seeds are delicious in salads, or sprinkle in some sesame seeds.

- Buy packs of mixed grains, such as quinoa, rice and barley, instead of just one type.

- Choose bags of mixed nuts instead of just eating almonds, for example.

- Replace some of the meat in bolognese sauce or shepherd's pie with lentils.

- Make mash with sweet potatoes or beans instead of always using white potatoes.

Before you know it, you'll be eating a whole rainbow of fruit, veg and spices – helping your microbiome to thrive.

THE GUT-BRAIN CONNECTION

We all know that saying 'Listen to your gut'. Well, turns out it's true. Your gut and your brain really are connected and your brain affects your gut health and vice versa. The brain is constantly sending messages all over the body, but the gut also talks back to the brain. One connection is through the vagus nerve – a complex nerve system that travels from the brain to the gut. The second way is through the neurotransmitters that your gut bacteria produce. A poor diet can lead to depression and mental health problems.

As we now know, the gut microbiome controls how well your immune system works. Initial research has shown that the gut microbiome stimulates the immune system's response to infection and supports the production of immune antibodies, which fight viruses. However, Linia says that research also shows that the bacteria don't do all the heavy lifting when it comes to interacting with the immune system: 'They have assistants: the metabolites they produce when they break down the fibre we eat. Chief among them are short-chain fatty acids (SCFAs) such as butyrates, which seem to be responsible for communicating our body's response to infection to our immune cells. Studies also show that these SCFAs help immune-modulating regulatory T-cells and reduce inflammation.'

poor diet can lead to mental health problems

VEGAN OR VEGETARIAN?

I don't eat red meat, just a little chicken and fish. I would say my diet is 90 per cent plant-based. It's clear from the research that we would be 100 per cent healthier if we ate more plant-based food. I asked Linia whether vegetarians or vegans are healthier than meat-eaters. Her response was that if you eat large amounts of meat, particularly processed meat, on a regular basis, that's not good for you. Whereas if you follow the Mediterranean example and have small portions of lean meat and fish as part of a very plant-based diet, then you derive more or less the same benefits as being vegetarian.

Science shows us that we need to eat more plants to be healthier. But in Linia's opinion, there's no current evidence to suggest that being vegan is better for your gut than being a vegetarian or being a meat-eater as long as you're following a balanced diet.

Linia added, 'If you're vegan and don't plan and organize your meals properly, avoiding animal products can lead to a reliance on unhealthy processed plant protein or refined carbohydrates. You really have to be on it. And what I'm seeing more and more of is processed vegan food. Now, if processed animal food is not healthy for us, what would make processed vegan food good for us? It's not. When we link this back to gut health, one of the things that has a negative effect on gut health is ingredients listed as emulsifiers. If you pick up a packet of pretty much any ultra-processed food, even processed vegan food, there are going to be emulsifiers there, and the fewer you eat of those, the better. The message is if you're a vegan who's eating in a traditional Indian dahl-and-rice type of way, fine. If you're eating lots of bread and processed vegan ready-meals and processed vegan cheese – that's not good news for your gut.'

Whether you're a vegan, vegetarian or omnivore, Linia stresses that quality is the key. Check labels and avoid things with a long list of unrecognizable ingredients and chemicals.

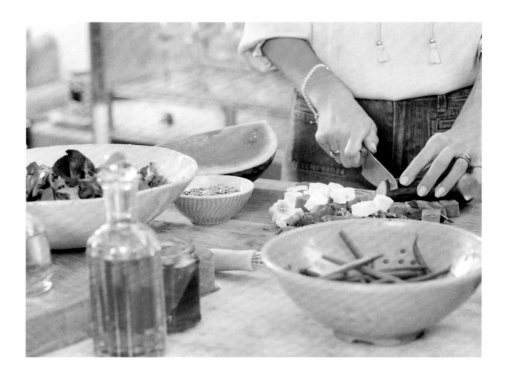

a healthy diet

So, what is a healthy diet? Basically, our food can be broken down into three groups and a healthy balanced diet should include all three:

+ carbohydrates

+ protein

+ fats

CARBOHYDRATES

Carbohydrates are often demonized, but they are essential for energy. There are two types of carbs – simple and complex. The simple carbs are the ones we can do very well without, such as white bread, cakes, biscuits and sweets. They are all low in fibre and can cause blood sugar spikes if eaten in excess.

Complex carbs, on the other hand, contain fibre and take longer to digest, so are much better for our blood sugar levels. They include vegetables, whole fruit (not juice), pulses and wholegrains.

PROTEIN

Protein helps us feel full and satisfied and is also vital to fuel growth and repair in the body. Animal sources of protein include meat, fish, eggs and dairy, but we can also get protein from plant sources, such as beans, nuts and seeds.

FATS

We need some fat in our diet for energy and to help us absorb nutrients. Saturated fat is found in fatty meat and dairy products. Healthier are the unsaturated fats – monounsaturated fats are found in foods such as nuts, seeds and olive oil, while oily fish and vegetable oils contain polyunsaturated fats. All kinds of fats are high in calories, so should be eaten in moderation.

THE MEDITERRANEAN DIET

We all want to enjoy our food and not be constantly fretting about what is on our plate, so the best solution is to adopt a sensible eating pattern that is delicious and healthy. Linia agrees that the Mediterranean way of eating, so often linked to good health outcomes, is a popular pattern and simple to follow.

The Mediterranean diet is high in fibre and low in sugar.

Key points are:

- plenty of vegetables and whole fruit
- nuts and seeds
- beans and lentils
- wholegrains
- fish, poultry and small amounts of lean meat
- olive oil
- some dairy, such as yoghurt and cheese

Raw versus cooked

Linia's take on this is that while with some vegetables you get more nutrients from raw than cooked, it doesn't work with everything. For instance, some beans contain proteins called lectins, which can cause digestive problems if not cooked. 'In general, we're not eating enough vegetables and fruit,' says Linia, 'so whether you eat them raw or cooked is much of a muchness. We just need to eat more of them.'

Eating the rainbow

We mentioned previously the importance of phytonutrients in plants for gut health. These nutrients, which have names such as flavonoids and polyphenols, all feed our gut microbiome, boost our immune system and reduce the risk of chronic diseases. An easy way to make sure you get a good range of these plant nutrients is to enjoy plant foods of different colours – orange carrots, red peppers, green cabbage, purple berries, yellow squash and so on. Research shows that flavonoids can contribute to brain health later in life and perhaps help to stave off conditions such as Alzheimer's.

Keep a check on sugar

Linia suggests keeping a careful limit on sugar intake, rather than banning or demonizing it. If you want a little jam or maple syrup on your crumpet, go ahead – but don't have more than 30g (1oz) a day. Too much added sugar is bad for your gut bacteria and so are artificial sweeteners if consumed habitually. If you want to make a cake, use sugar and real butter, just don't do it every day.

too much added sugar is bad for your gut bacteria

Fruit

Always eat whole fruit, not just juice, as the fibre helps slow the digestive process so you don't get a sugar rush. Fruit contains natural sugars. In whole fruit, the sugar is bound within the structure of the fruit (intrinsic sugar) so when you eat fruit whole, it hits your bloodstream more slowly than sugary food and drinks.

Interestingly, juice only counts as one of your five-a-day no matter how much of it you drink. The reason for this is that the process of juicing fruit releases the sugar from the cells' walls and that is why fruit juice contains free sugars. In addition, juicing loses most of the valuable fibre found in the whole fruit. Therefore, recommendations are that we limit the intake of fruit juice and shop-bought smoothies to 150ml (5fl oz) per day. As a point of reference, one glass (200ml/7fl oz) of 100 per cent pressed apple juice contains 5 teaspoons of sugar (20g/¾oz), which almost clocks up your daily free sugar intake for the day.

The good news is that homemade smoothies/blended juices, using the whole fruit or vegetable, can count as two portions, depending on the amount of pulp (fibre) they contain. Blenders grind, mix or emulsify all of your ingredients together, so what you put into a blender is what you consume.

Pasta

Linia spends half her life in Italy and knows how much the Italians love their pasta, but they don't overeat it nor do they they overcook it. Pasta can have a high glycaemic index (the glycaemic index (GI) is basically how quickly the sugar is released from carbohydrates into your blood). The higher the GI of a food, the greater the effect on your blood sugar. Italians eat their pasta al dente – still with a little bite to it – which means it has a lower GI than very well-cooked pasta, so is better for your blood sugar levels. And even better – if you cook pasta, let it cool and eat it in a pasta salad. This creates something called resistance starch, which is a type of fibre your gut bacteria love.

Italians eat pasta al dente which has a lower GI

Nuts and seeds

Nuts and seeds contain omega-3 – polyunsaturated fats – which are heart-healthy and can reduce inflammation. Ideally, eat them raw though – not roasted, toasted or salted. The roasting process changes the structure of the fat. It's fine to eat roasted nuts occasionally but not as a regular thing.

Meat

I've never liked red meat – it makes me think of chewing a body! I'm fine with chicken or fish just not red meat, although I do still cook it for the family very occasionally. Left to his own devices, my husband would probably be happy eating meat every day – his idea of heaven is a giant rare steak – but all I see on that plate is something that will raise your cholesterol and clog up your arteries. Not to mention the fact that meat stays undigested in your colon for ages!

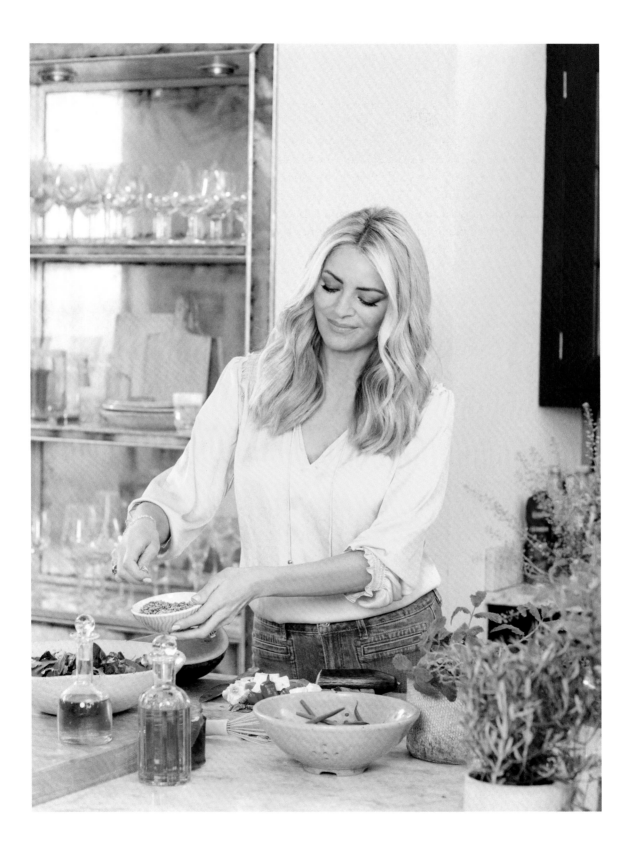

The World Health Organization suggests limiting red meat intake to 350g (12oz) a week and of that total, very little processed red meat. According to Linia, processed meat is the really bad stuff – anything that has nitrates and other chemicals added to it, such as bacon and ham. There is a clear link between processed meat and cancer, so the less you have of it, the better. If you keep red meat to the recommended limits, it doesn't necessarily have an impact on cancer. But if you cook it on a barbecue, the risk increases if done habitually. When you cook meat at a high temperature on a barbecue, it produces something called heterocyclic amines, which are the burnt bits that smell so delicious. And too many of these can start the process of cancer in the bowel.

it's always better to spread your protein throughout the day

'The part of your bowel that digests protein is called the terminal ileum and is not that long,' Linia says, 'so we can't digest a lot of protein at once and this is why it's always better to spread your protein throughout the day. The reason why too much meat can cause cancer is because if you're habitually eating too much red meat, the bowel tries to do as much digestion as it can, but then bits that it can't digest go into the large bowel. The large bowel's job is not to digest and so over time that increases your risk of getting cancer because you're exposing it to all these carcinogens that are not digested. So that's why if you just look at the dietary patterns of people who eat too much meat, they have higher levels of colon cancer.'

But Linia points out that meat does contain valuable nutrients. In a recent dietary survey in the UK, teenage girls were shown to be lacking in iron and zinc – and where are those found? In red meat. So her view is not to totally avoid meat – unless you want to – but to have it in moderation. Perhaps when making a meat sauce or a chilli, try reducing the amount of meat and bulk it up with beans and lentils. That way you're getting the best of both worlds.

Dairy

Again, Linia agrees, it's a question of balance. Yes, dairy foods contain saturated fat, but they are also one of the best sources of calcium and they contain protein. In Linia's view, it's a no to drinking copious quantities of milk once you're over 2 years old but having some in your tea and coffee is fine. And cheese and yoghurt are less of a problem than cream or butter. They are fermented foods so contain probiotics, which are basically live bacteria and good for gut health. In some regions, such as Korea, they eat lots of fermented foods like kimchi, but in the West live yoghurt is probably the easiest option for most people, so go for it, Linia advises, and opt for the full-fat version. Cheese too, although it's high in fat so control your portion size – a thumb-sized piece a day is fine.

As to plant milks, for women Linia recommends soya as that has the highest amount of phytoestrogens. As we get older, our oestrogen levels drop so having more of the plant-based oestrogens is helpful – unless you're at a high risk of breast cancer, in which case the message is different. Oat milk is the most sustainable of the plant milks, but it's lower in protein and contains lower amounts of phytoestrogens. She suggests ringing the changes between regular milk and plant milks rather than getting hooked on one type.

Oils

Different oils vary in their smoking point. Once the oil gets so hot it starts to smoke,.the structure of the oil changes which can result in it losing some of its nutritional value and giving food an unpleasant taste.

Linia advises using olive oil for salads and for sautéing at low temperatures but not for cooking at high temperatures. For other purposes, like roasting potatoes, for example, use lard or goose fat, and for stir-fries, coconut oil is good – but not too much of it.

the next step to gut health

Getting your nutrition right is a journey, Linia says. First off, she wants to see people getting the basics right – are they eating plenty of vegetables and fruit and a good variety? Are they eating balanced meals? Are they drinking enough water? Once those are in place, it's time to think about other issues, such as the quality of food, how and when you eat and potential problems.

GO FOR ORGANIC?

Has the chicken you cook had a chance to run around? Has the cow your beef comes from been able to feed on grass? If budget allows, it's certainly worth opting for free-range chicken and grass-fed beef. Looking at fruit and vegetables, Linia warns that some, such as strawberries and tomatoes, are grown using particularly high levels of chemicals, so it's good to go for organic or bio for those, if possible. (Bio products are not totally organic but are produced with a much lower level of chemicals.)

MINDFUL EATING

During the mid-nineties, I lived and worked in France for a number of years. The dietary habits there were a startling revelation to me. I could not believe the Parisians I was working with stopped for several hours to eat a three-course lunch – with wine served alongside the water. Alcohol at lunchtime, at work – nuts! It wasn't for me – I would just feel like having a sleep after such a long lunch – but what struck me was the dedication, the near reverence, for the ritual of sitting down to savour a meal. In France, lunch is an almost sacred experience and one that should never ever be rushed.

That just wasn't what I was used to and for a while, I stuck to my old 'eat-on-the-run' habits. Sometimes I'd be walking through Paris eating a baguette and complete strangers would tap me on the shoulder and ask if I wanted to sit down. They were visibly worried about me eating on the go. And Linia agrees that it is not only about what you eat, but how you eat, that's important. Eating in a rush doesn't help your gut at all. If you're not chewing enough, you're not going to digest your food properly, so you're not giving your body the best start.

If you eat in front of the TV, on the move or at your desk, you're less likely to appreciate your food; you're then less likely to notice when you're full and to keep on eating – and possibly overeat. Far better to sit down at the table, relax and think about what you are eating and appreciate it. Where possible, enjoy eating as a social activity – a chance to share good food and conversation with family or friends in a relaxed setting.

FASTING

It used to be thought that missing meals slowed down your metabolism and that was why yo-yo dieting was not good for you and messed up your system. But around the same time as the realizations about the importance of gut health, along came the whole theory of intermittent fasting. The research was done using mice first, and mice who had a third less of their calories for the day seemed to live longer. And not only did they live longer, but their metabolic health was better, so they were not getting diseases like heart disease, cancers and auto-immune conditions.

Why is fasting good for us? Well, it basically allows our body time to rest. It gives your gut bacteria time to start doing their thing and to repair the gut. But Linia has found that the benefits of either 5:2 fasting or eating within an 8-hour window aren't the same for everyone: 'For men and for post-menopausal women, the fasting regime can work well. But women of reproductive age do not benefit in the same way and that is because what drives us fundamentally is our ability to reproduce. We have something called the hypothalamic axis which connects the brain to the organs that produce various hormones. In that axis are certain proteins – neuropeptides – that are sensitive to energy intake and one of them is called kisspeptin. Women have a higher amount of kisspeptin than men, which means we're much more sensitive to energy regulation. So, if I was to do high-intensity exercise while in a fasted state and make that a habit, I would start getting frustrated after a while because I wouldn't lose fat. In fact, I might gain a little fat and lose some muscle because my body would ultimately be trying to protect my reproductive function. That is why women produce more stress hormones when they fast than men do, and the stress hormones then have a negative impact in terms of body composition.'

But some degree of fasting is beneficial, so for women of reproductive age, Linia advises maximizing your overnight fast. Leave 12 hours between dinner and breakfast, but then make sure you eat breakfast. This should allow your gut time to rest and repair without stressing the body.

leave 12 hours between dinner and breakfast, but then make sure you eat breakfast

BALANCING BLOOD SUGAR

Sugary foods and simple carbohydrates, as we know, cause your blood sugar to rise. When you wake up in the morning, a hormone called cortisol is released and this helps you get up and get going. Ideally, eat a balanced breakfast with some wholegrain, fibre-rich carbs and some protein to help regulate the amount of cortisol released through the day. If you eat refined cereal and fruit juice, this provides very little fibre and just sugar, sugar, sugar. Your blood sugar levels will then shoot up and crash a couple of hours later. Have a look at the breakfast recipes in this book (see pages 53–65) for some healthier ways to start the day, with dishes containing plenty of fibre and protein.

If you balance your blood sugar successfully, the world is a happy place but if too much sugar is released into your system, your body perceives that as a stress and your gut suffers.

HYDRATION IS A FUNDAMENTAL NEED FOR OUR BODY BECAUSE WE ARE 75 PER CENT WATER.

DRINK WATER

Hydration is a fundamental need for our body because we are 75 per cent water. If we don't hydrate, our appetite is not regulated and when you get that mid-afternoon slump, it's more likely to be thirst than hunger. Linia recommends drinking about 1.5 litres (2½ pints) a day for a woman, and 2 litres (3½ pints) for a man on average, but obviously this varies depending on what you are eating, activity levels and so on. Drinking water before a meal can also help you feel fuller – that's why soup can be good as a starter if you struggle with appetite control.

A LITTLE WINE OR NOT?

There have long been claims that some alcohol is good for us, but the evidence is, Linia says, that it does not really do much for our health.

Apparently, alcohol is most beneficial at the age of about 50, when heart disease becomes the biggest risk factor for death. Studies have shown that a glass of something can chill you out a bit and helps reduce that risk. Linia says that if we're thinking about gut health, the best drink is probably red wine because it contains phytochemicals – the stuff that gives the grapes their colour – but in general, the actual alcohol itself is not good for your gut bacteria. Her advice is to enjoy some alcohol if you want to but keep within recommended units for a week. However, there are other considerations. If, for example, you are at high risk of breast cancer, alcohol increases that risk so is best avoided. And, of course, alcohol is high in calories. Linia tells me she works with people who eat a wonderfully healthy diet but then go out and drink a couple of bottles of wine in an evening. That's a huge number of calories – your gut suffers, your muscles suffer and you feel bad the next day. So, yet again, moderation is key and don't use alcohol as a crutch to allow you to destress. You might think it is helping but actually it is a depressant and can make things worse.

don't use alcohol as a crutch to allow you to destress

gut
problems

ULTRA-PROCESSED FOOD

More and more research is showing that a high intake of ultra-processed foods is bad for our gut and bad for health. It can increase inflammation in the body, cause us to become overweight and potentially lead to health problems. That's not to say that a bag of crisps or a chocolate biscuit once in a while is going to ruin your life. I'll allow myself a chocolate bar at four o'clock if I want it because otherwise I'm going to think about it too much, and it's going to become a thing. I'm not into playing mind games with myself about the food that I consume and what I can and can't eat. It's all about moderation, that's always been my mantra.

People have done experiments greatly increasing their intake of ultra-processed foods for a limited period and the results have been detrimental to health, so all the evidence is to keep these foods to a small percentage of your overall intake. Linia advises cooking your meals from scratch as far as possible, using fresh ingredients, and limiting ready-meals and prepared foods. For example, instead of putting a jar of ready-made tomato sauce on your pasta, make your own with fresh tomatoes. Instead of buying a pack of sugary breakfast cereal, mix up some muesli with oats, nuts and seeds. You'll do yourself and your gut a big favour. But, when life gets hectic and you do reach out for pre-prepared meals, just make sure you read the labels and think about how you can add veggies to the meal to make it more balanced.

cook your
meals from
scratch when
possible

Eat well 70 to 80 per cent of the time, with a diet of fresh, whole foods and a good variety of fruit and vegetables, and what you eat the other 20 to 30 per cent doesn't matter as much. Again, a little of what you fancy does you good.

INFLAMMATION

Inflammation in the body is linked to all sorts of illnesses. It can be caused by stress but also has much to do with what we eat and our gut. A good gut microbiome lessens inflammation, but a bad diet packed with sugary and high-saturated fat or processed-fat foods and additives can build up and cause inflammation in the gut, which then has a knock-on effect on the rest of the body.

+   Added sugar, ultra-processed food and excess alcohol
    – all increase inflammation.

+   Wholegrains, omega-3-rich foods and colourful vegetables
    – all reduce inflammation.

OMEGA-3/OMEGA-6

Omega-3 and omega-6 are essential fatty acids. The body needs them, but we can't produce them, so we must get them from our food. Omega-3 is anti-inflammatory while omega-6 is pro-inflammatory, and you need a balance. For example, if you cut your finger, it's the inflammation process that enables you to bleed and then the anti-inflammatory process that forms a scab, so you don't bleed to death. A healthy ratio for our body is two to three times omega-6 to omega-3.

But nowadays, Linia says, we are not getting enough omega-3 due to changes linked to the food system. Foods that used to be high in omega-3 are less so now, and we don't eat enough oily fish (rich in omega-3) while omega-6, found in refined vegetable oils, is everywhere. Pick up almost any kind of processed food and refined vegetable oil will be listed in the ingredients, so the ratio for many of us is way off-kilter. Linia finds that the only people she meets with a good omega-3/omega-6 ratio are those who are avid fish eaters or who take a supplement.

Foods high in omega-3 include:

+ flaxseed oil

+ chia seeds

+ oily fish, such as mackerel, herring, trout, sardines

+ walnuts

+ seaweed

The recommendation is to have two portions a week of oily fish for omega-3, but even that might not be enough. Linia tells me that she is seeing such high levels of inflammation in some patients that they need more than the recommended intake of omega-3 to balance things out. For those people, supplements may be the answer. Another concern she has is that our seas are now so contaminated that there can be high levels of contamination in fish – and the bigger the fish, the more they might contain. She advises eating fish but choosing the smaller varieties more often, such as mackerel, sardines and anchovies. Mussels are another good source of omega-3 and also zinc, which is good for our skin, and they are sustainable.

FOOD INTOLERANCES

There is some evidence that food allergies and food sensitivities may be linked to imbalances in the makeup of your gut microbiome. Unlike food allergies or food sensitivities, food intolerances don't involve your immune system. For most people, food intolerances cause digestive problems with symptoms in your gut like bloating, gas, diarrhoea and constipation. For some people, food intolerances can cause other issues, including headaches and skin reactions.

The main causes of food intolerances are:

+ lactose – from dairy products such as milk, cheese, butter and yoghurt

+ wheat

+ gluten – in rye, wheat, barley, beer

Food intolerances, like lactose intolerance, can be genetic and run in your family. Or they may be related to other conditions, such as irritable bowel syndrome (IBS). In recent research, they have been linked to taking long courses of antibiotics. Over-exposure to foods may also play a role. For example, modern farming methods mean that wheat now contains more gluten and gliadin (a component of gluten) than it used to, so we're seeing more intolerance. And if you're eating cereal for breakfast, a sandwich for lunch and pasta for supper, you're exposing yourself more to the food that causes that intolerance.

Food intolerances don't always have a single, easily identifiable cause. If you feel you are suffering from an intolerance, try to record your symptoms and what you eat to get a fuller picture. Linia advises caution in giving up whole food groups without guidance. If you're worried about a food reaction you're experiencing, it's important to talk to a trusted healthcare professional before you restrict what you eat.

IRRITABLE BOWEL SYNDROME

IBS is a gastrointestinal (GI) disorder characterized by irregular bowel habits (diarrhoea and/or constipation), bloating, flatulence and cramps. The exact cause of IBS is still unknown. Factors that may contribute to developing IBS include impaired gut–brain communication, stress, psychological conditions (such as anxiety or depression) and altered gut bacteria.

Various factors affect or worsen IBS, including your mental state and dietary factors. Linia emphasizes the importance of IBS treatment being holistic, including mind management as well as dietary intervention. 'For people with IBS, digestive reaction to high-FODMAP foods can be one cause of food intolerance symptoms. FODMAP stands for fermentable oligosaccharides, disaccharides, monosaccharides and polyols, which are types of sugar found in specific foods. IBS is complex but a low-FODMAP diet has been shown to improve symptoms. If you think you have IBS, it is essential to seek help from a health professional. The FODMAP diet is not one to do on your own with the help of Google. It is best followed with the help of a dietitian.'

IBS has been linked with leaky gut syndrome (increased intestinal permeability). However, although the body of research is growing, there is still a lot to learn about increased intestinal permeability and

IBS treatment should be holistic

how it contributes to conditions like IBS. Linia says that what we do know is that the gut has an intestinal barrier: 'This barrier allows the "good stuff", like nutrients, gut bacteria, fluid and electrolytes, to cross into the gut and acts as a stop to prevent the "bad stuff", like toxins or pathogenic bacteria, from entering. Leaky gut basically means that some of the "bad stuff" enters the gut more easily and is associated with a variety of conditions, such as coeliac disease, inflammatory bowel disease, food intolerances and chronic fatigue. Although there is a growing body of research on leaky gut, there is still a lot we don't know, for example, the exact causes.'

there is still a lot we don't know about leaky gut syndrome

'We do know that there are factors that can increase intestinal permeability, such as a low fibre diet, habitual intake of ultra-processed foods that are high in added sugar and refined or saturated fat, excessive alcohol consumption, antibiotic use and even chronic overuse of non-steroid anti-inflammatory drugs (NSAIDs), such as ibuprofen.'

ASSESSING YOUR OWN GUT HEALTH

'People are always asking me what's normal in terms of bowel habits,' says Linia. 'But the answer is there is no normal. Some people go several times every day; others every couple of days. But one thing that is becoming clear is that the time it takes for food to transit through your gut is a good indicator of gut health.'

It turns out there's an easy test for this that you can do yourself at home and it's part of a major study on gut health. It's called the blue poop test. Check online and you will find a recipe for making muffins and adding some blue food dye (joinzoe.com/bluepoop). You eat these and see how long it takes for the blue poo to appear. You then input your data on the research site and get some very useful info on the health of your gut. Plus when else would you get to do blue poo?!

We know that we all bloat a little bit after a meal, that's normal, but chronic bloating when you start to look like you're six months pregnant, frequent indigestion or alternating diarrhoea and constipation are all signs that you've got poor gut health and maybe you need to take action.

LINIA'S ROUTE TO GOOD GUT HEALTH

Don't go low on carbs

To maintain a high diversity of gut bacteria (the aim of the game), you need to ensure that you include carbs in the form of wholegrains, fruit and vegetables. Within these types of carbohydrates are types of fibre that are known to have a 'prebiotic' effect. That means they feed the 'good' bacteria, therefore enriching your gut microbiota. Current dietary guidelines recommend that we eat about 30g of fibre per day, but research reveals that most of us are only eating about 19g. Fibre is underrated yet, in fact, it is a Holy Grail nutrient. If you can increase the amount you eat, it will not only benefit how your gut functions, but will also have a positive impact on your waistline, your heart and pretty much every organ in your body.

ACTION

+ Gradually increase the amount of fibre in your diet to give your body time to adjust.

+ Opt for wholegrain carbohydrates wherever possible.

Don't always eat the same thing

Are you a routine kind of person when it comes to food? If so, then the chances are that the diversity of your diet is low. As recent research suggests, we should be aiming to eat at least 30 different plant-based foods each week, not just fixating on eating the same things all the time. If you regularly eat wild rice, try another grain like spelt, farro, quinoa or buckwheat. Better still, buy a mixed grain. The same goes for tins of beans. It's great if you always add a tin of chickpeas to your weekly shop, but how about swapping this for a four-bean mix instead? Try lentil, bean or wholewheat versions of pasta. Buy in-season fruit and veg, which means you won't always be eating the same things.

ACTION

+ Aim for 30 different types of plant-based foods per week.

+ Each week, add in a new type of vegetable, fruit, nut, seed and wholegrain.

Cut out junk food

Not surprisingly, our gut bacteria do not thrive on junk food. Recent research has shown neither do they like you to include artificial sweeteners in your diet in large amounts or as a daily routine. Although diet versions may help reduce your calorie intake, based on evidence from animal studies they may destroy the diversity of your gut microbiome. Whether you're better off having sugar instead of sweeteners will depend on a number of things, such as your medical history and your weight. However, this research implied that if you want to indulge in something sweet, you may be better off opting for the product that has sugar in it, rather than artificial sweeteners. However, this is not a green flag to eat your way through a bag of sweets! As unsexy as it sounds, it's all about balance.

ACTION

+ Read the labels and see which products contain artificial sweeteners.

Up the fermented foods

The process of fermenting involves bacteria and yeast, so increasing your intake of fermented foods has a positive impact on your gut microbiome. Fermented foods can provide health benefits beyond basic nutrition and scientists are still investigating exactly how they affect our bodies and health. Some studies have linked the intake of fermented foods to a reduced risk of cardiovascular disease, type 2 diabetes and better gut health.

Kefir is one of the fermented foods that has the most research behind it. It contains 20 different types of bacteria and yeast, making it a great addition to your diet. Other gut-friendly fermented foods include bio-live yoghurt, kimchi, sauerkraut, miso, tempeh and sourdough bread. If you suffer from irritable bowel syndrome, then be aware that many fermented foods are also high in FODMAPs, which can trigger gut symptoms.

ACTION

+ Aim to include at least one fermented food in your diet each day.

+ Always opt for bio-live yoghurt as this will contain live bacteria cultures.

Work up a sweat

The more you move, the happier your gut bacteria are. This is particularly true when it comes to some cardio work. When the microbiome of professional athletes is compared to that of normal sedentary people, the results always show that the microbiomes of the athletes are far more diverse than average. In a number of studies on other animals, the results also show that exercise induces positive changes in the gut microbiota that are different to the effects induced by diet. The good bacteria that seem to flourish with exercise are Lactobacillus, Bifidobacterium and B. coccoides–E. rectale group. However, as with everything, it's about moderation. Don't over-exercise, as too much can be detrimental to your gut.

ACTION

+ Think of ways you can move more. Have a look at page 186 for some great exercise ideas – even some you can do while waiting for the kettle to boil!

Sleep on it

Good-quality, refreshing sleep is good for your gut. More and more research is showing that the better we sleep, the more our gut microbiome flourishes and vice versa. The sleep–gut link is complex and a recent study showed that after just two nights of sleep deprivation there were significant decreases in the types of beneficial bacteria. Other research has shown that poor sleep may also raise the risk of experiencing gastrointestinal issues like IBS. A study on rats found that when prebiotics (fibre-containing foods that feed your microbiome) were given to sleep-deprived and stressed rats, it helped them restore a normal sleep pattern and get more good-quality REM sleep.

ACTION

+ If you have had stress-related sleep disruption, then load up on prebiotic foods like garlic, onions, leeks, asparagus, mushrooms, bananas and blueberries.

Chill out

When you're stressed out, your body releases stress hormones, which in turn cause your immune system to release inflammatory substances called cytokines. These send inflammation messages to all parts of your body, including your gut bacteria. Over a long period of time, this can have a negative effect, increasing the leakiness of your gut and also causing an unbalanced microbiome. Learning to chill out is key to keeping your microbiome balanced and diverse and, if you are already experiencing gut health issues, will help to heal your gut.

ACTION

+ Carve out a little chill out you-time every day. Try some breathing exercises that you'll find on pages 168–173.

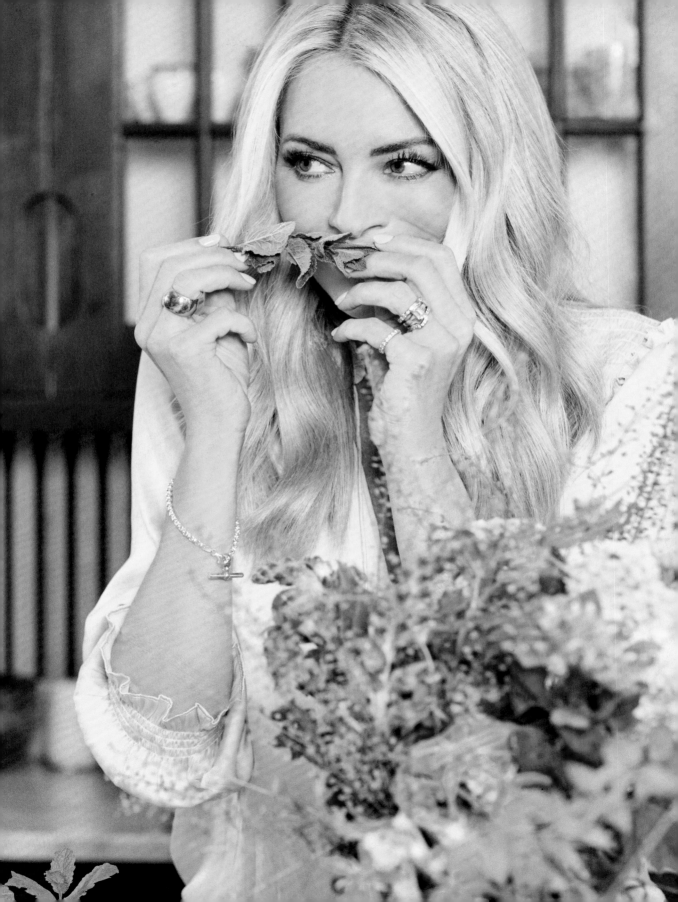

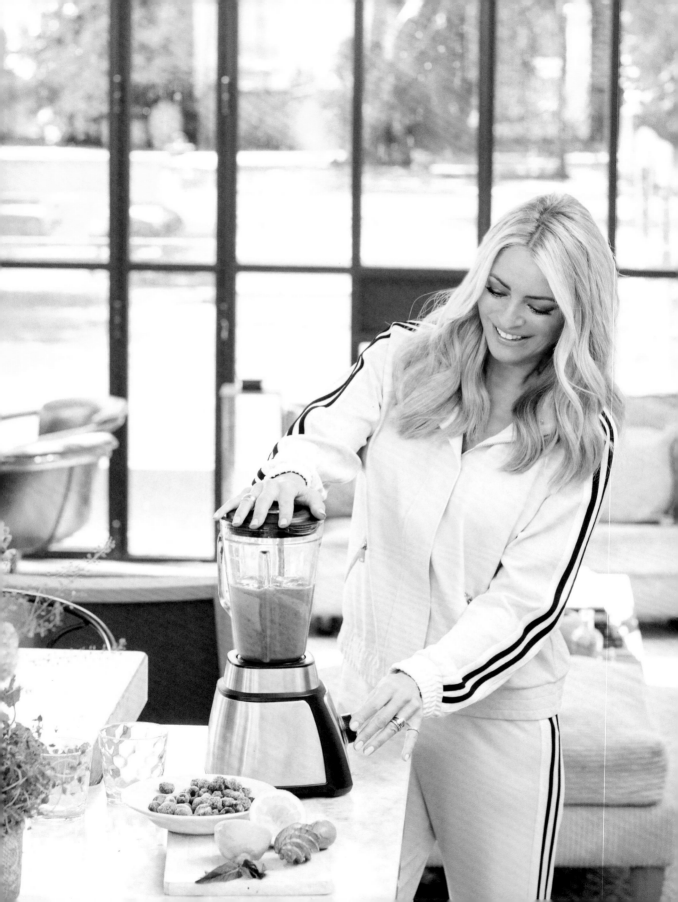

BREAKFAST
+ BRUNCH

Kickstart your metabolism

Blissful Breakfast Sundaes

Recent research shows that having 30 different plant-based foods a week boosts your gut health and this sundae, with all the fruit, nuts and seeds, gets you off to a good start. It's a very easy-going recipe that you can change to suit your taste and store cupboard. Try adding a little finely chopped crystallized ginger, a couple of spoonfuls of dried mango or pineapple or some flaked coconut.

PREP 10 MINS
COOK LESS THAN 10 MINS
SERVES 4

FOR THE MUESLI MIX (ENOUGH FOR 8 PORTIONS)

25g (1oz) butter or coconut oil
50g (1¾oz) oats
50g (1¾oz) mixed nuts, roughly chopped (I used flaked almonds, pecans, hazelnuts, Brazils)
a pinch of salt
50g (1¾oz) mixed seeds (I used a mixture of pumpkin, sunflower, sesame)
¼ tsp ground cinnamon
¼ tsp ground cardamom
2 tbsp honey

TO ASSEMBLE

600g (1lb 5oz) Greek yoghurt
250g (9oz) strawberries, hulled and halved if large
250g (9oz) raspberries
250g (9oz) blueberries
honey, for drizzling
a few mint leaves

First, make the muesli mix. Melt the butter or oil in a large frying pan. Add the oats and nuts with a pinch of salt and stir over a medium-low heat until you can smell that they are lightly toasted. This will take 3 to 4 minutes. Add the seeds and spices. Cook for another minute, then drizzle in the honey and continue to stir-fry until well combined. The mixture will be very lightly browned with a bit of crunch. Leave to cool.

To assemble the sundaes, take four bowls or sundae glasses. Put some of the muesli mix in the base, followed by a couple of tablespoons of yoghurt, then add a mixture of fruit. Repeat the layers, then drizzle over some honey and garnish with a few mint leaves.

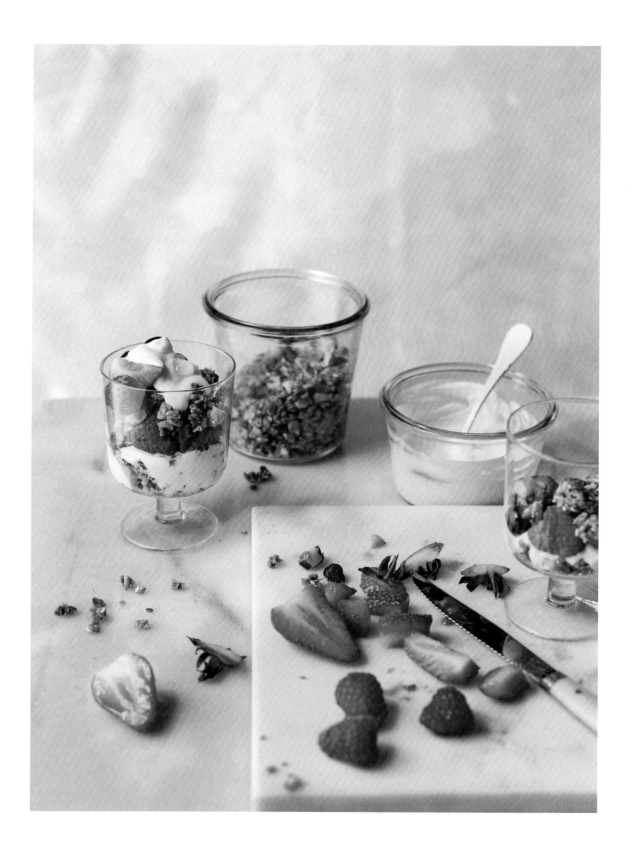

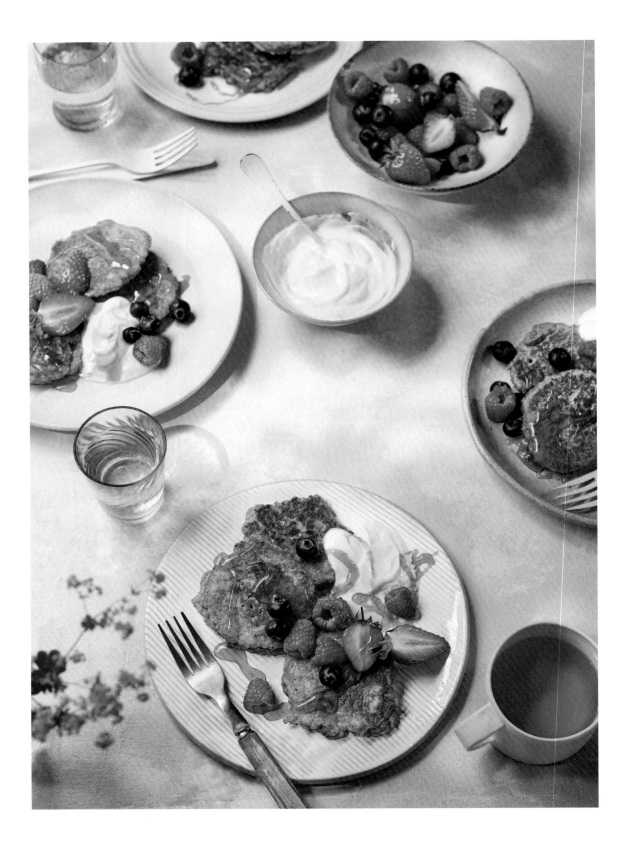

Bouncing Banana Pancakes

So named because you'll literally bounce with energy after eating them, thanks to that lovely banana and oat combo. These pancakes are a regular for breakfast in my house and the number-one weekend request from my girls and their sleepover guests. Sometimes I use Ready Brek instead of oats – it makes the prep even easier. I do find that the pancakes can be quite fragile though, so best not to make them too big and take care when flipping – don't go too wild!

If using oats, put in a food processor and whiz until they still have some texture, but are much flourier in consistency. Mix with the baking powder, cinnamon and nutmeg, if using, as well as a pinch of salt.

Blend the bananas, eggs and yoghurt together, then mix with the oat mixture and the protein powder or seeds, if using.

Melt a knob of butter in a large frying pan. Put small ladlefuls of the mixture (around 2 tablespoons per pancake) into the frying pan and cook on a medium heat. Don't have the heat too high or the underside will burn before the pancakes are set. When they are firm enough on the underside – 3 to 4 minutes – flip over and cook the top side for another couple of minutes. Transfer to a plate and keep warm while you cook the rest. You should end up with 12 to 16 pancakes.

Serve with more yoghurt, a drizzle of honey or maple syrup and a few berries.

PREP 10 MINUTES
COOK ABOUT 20 MINUTES
SERVES 4

125g (4½oz) oats or oatmeal
  (e.g. Ready Brek)
2 tsp baking powder
½ tsp ground cinnamon
  (optional)
a few gratings of nutmeg
  (optional)
a pinch of salt
2 bananas
2 eggs
75g (3oz) thick live yoghurt
1 tbsp protein powder
  (optional)
1 tbsp milled flax seeds
  (optional)
A few knobs of butter

TO SERVE
yoghurt
honey or maple syrup
berries

Bursting Blueberries French Toast

PREP 10 MINUTES
COOK 15 MINUTES
SERVES 4

3 eggs
150ml (5fl oz) milk
1 tbsp maple syrup
¼ tsp ground cinnamon
a pinch of salt
25g (1oz) butter
8 slices of brioche, halved
  if you like

FOR THE BLUEBERRY COMPOTE
250g (9oz) blueberries, fresh
  or frozen
a squeeze of lime juice
2 tsp honey

TO SERVE
yoghurt or crème fraîche

This is a quick-and-easy treat that my family loves for a lazy late Sunday brunch. Blueberries are often called a superfood as they contain good amounts of several vitamins, including vitamin C, so I always like to have some in the freezer. Frozen berries are just as nutritious as fresh – and often cheaper! You could also sprinkle some sesame seeds on top of the French toast – they're a great source of calcium – and maybe some extra cinnamon or a light dusting of icing sugar for a touch of decadence.

First, make the compote. Put the blueberries in a small saucepan with the lime juice, honey and a splash of water (around 3 tablespoons). Heat gently just until the blueberries burst and create their own sauce – a minute or two if using frozen blueberries, a few more if using fresh. Keep warm.

To make the French toast, put the eggs, milk, maple syrup and cinnamon into a bowl with a pinch of salt and whisk thoroughly.

Heat half the butter in a large frying pan. Dip half the slices of brioche in the egg mixture, making sure they soak right through, but not letting them get so saturated they will fall apart. Gently scrape off any excess and add to the frying pan. Fry the brioche over a medium heat until golden brown and set on the underside, then flip over and cook for another few minutes.

Remove from the pan and keep warm, then repeat with the remaining butter, egg mixture and brioche.

Serve the brioche with spoonfuls of the compote and a dollop of yoghurt or crème fraîche, if you like.

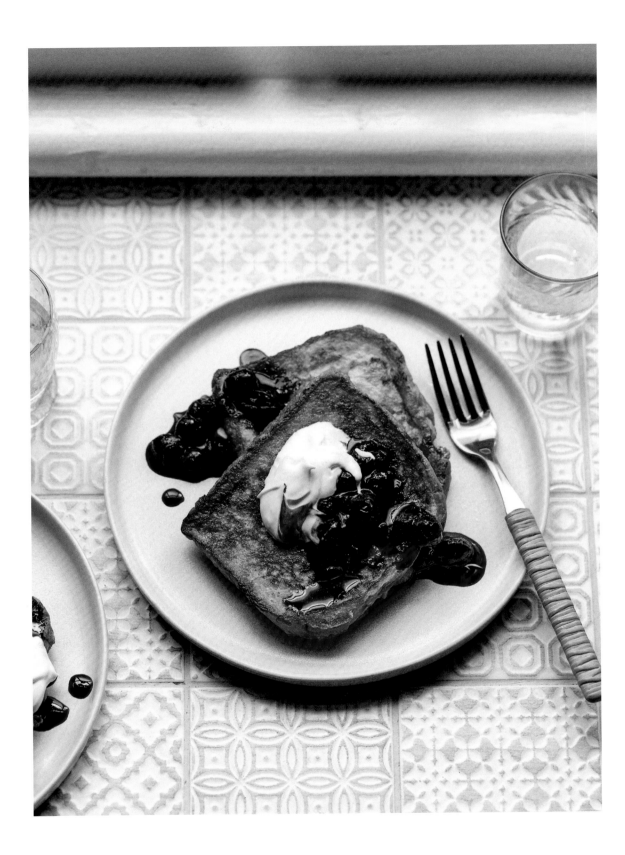

Take-your-pick Omelettes

PREP 10 MINUTES

COOK 10 MINUTES

BASIC OMELETTE SERVES 1,
FILLINGS ARE ENOUGH
FOR 4 OMELETTES APIECE

FOR THE BASIC OMELETTE

3 eggs, beaten

a knob of butter

salt and black pepper

FOR THE MUSHROOM FILLING

15g (½oz) butter

300g (10½oz) mushrooms,
   sliced

2 large garlic cloves, finely
   chopped

leaves from a sprig of tarragon,
   finely chopped (optional)

**FOR THE CABBAGE, CARROT
AND KIMCHI FILLING**

1 tbsp olive oil

150g (5½oz) cabbage, finely
   shredded

1 large carrot, coarsely grated

100g (3½oz) kimchi, roughly
   chopped

Eggs are a great source of protein, and an omelette makes a speedy, filling meal for breakfast or any time of day. A plain one is delicious, but I've suggested some of my favourite fillings to try. You could also just add grated cheese, shredded ham or fresh herbs to the basic recipe. Some smoked mackerel or trout would be a tasty addition to the spinach version for extra protein. Pictured overleaf.

First, make any of the fillings you want to use and prepare any optional extras.

To make the mushroom filling, heat the butter in a large frying pan. Add the mushrooms and season with salt and pepper. Fry until the mushrooms have cooked down and are glossy. Add the garlic and tarragon, if using, and cook for another couple of minutes.

To make the cabbage, carrot and kimchi filling, heat the oil in a frying pan. Add the cabbage and carrot and season with salt and pepper. Sauté, stirring regularly, until the cabbage has collapsed down and softened. Stir in the kimchi and simmer to make sure the mixture is relatively dry. Remove from the heat.

To make the wilted spinach, wash the spinach thoroughly and put it in a saucepan. Heat, pushing down with a wooden spoon, until it wilts down, then strain over a colander and roughly chop. Add a squeeze of lemon juice and a fine grating of nutmeg, if using.

To make each omelette, break the eggs into a bowl and beat thoroughly so they are well broken up. Season with salt and pepper.

Heat up your omelette pan and when it is hot, add the butter. It should immediately start to melt and foam. As soon as it is completely melted, pour in the eggs and swirl so they coat the entire base of the pan. Using a fork, keep pulling the eggs in from the side to the centre, swirling the pan as you do so, so the space created is filled up with the remaining raw egg. Continue to do this until the omelette is no longer runny. Leave for another minute or so until it is almost set.

Add your choice of filling, plus any optional extras, in a line along the middle. Flip one side of the omelette over the filling, then roll it over so the filling is completely encased. Slide onto a plate and serve.

FOR THE WILTED SPINACH FILLING
450g (1lb) bag of baby spinach
a squeeze of lemon juice
a grating of nutmeg (optional)

OPTIONAL EXTRAS
grated cheese
flaked hot smoked fish (e.g. smoked mackerel or trout)
finely shredded turkey ham
any herbs (tarragon, basil, chives, dill)

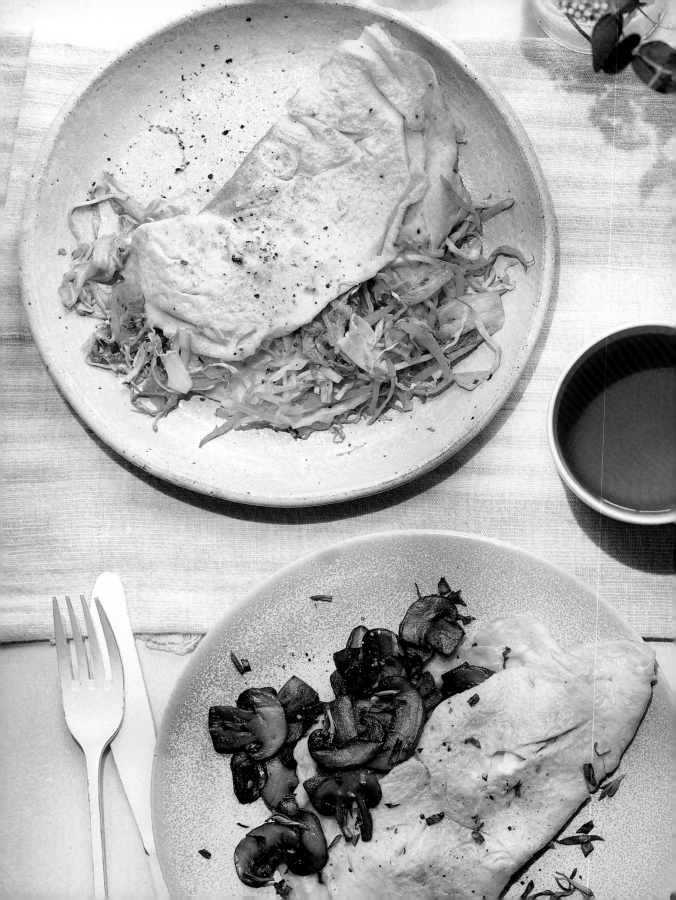

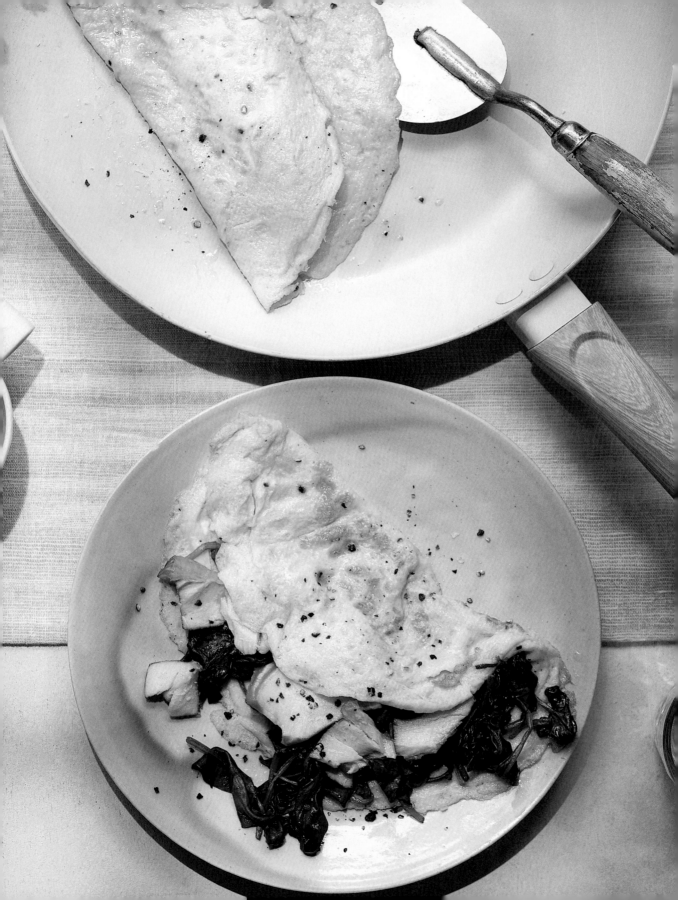

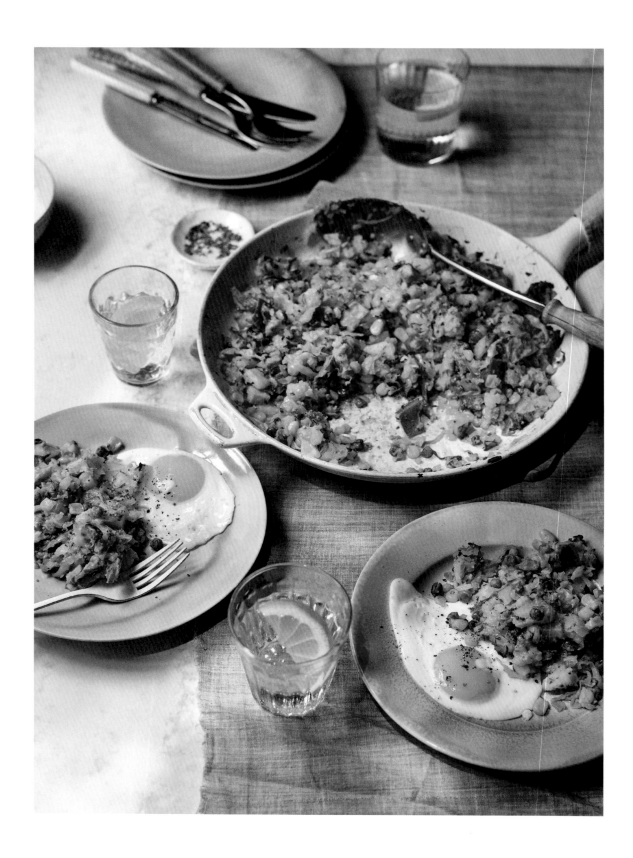

Banging Bubble + Squeak

I hate wasting food as it makes neither economic nor ecological sense, and a bubble and squeak is a great way of using up leftover mash or any other cooked veg. When cooking a hash from scratch as here, I like to leave the skins on the potatoes as much of their nutritional value is just under the skin. I find steaming them gives the best result, as the flesh will be drier – sweet potatoes in particular can get rather waterlogged. You don't have to add the spices but they make this dish pop with flavour and they're excellent for gut health.

PREP 15 MINUTES
COOK ABOUT 35 MINUTES
SERVES 4

400g (14oz) sweet potatoes, well-scrubbed and cut into chunks

300g (10½oz) floury potatoes, well-scrubbed and cut into chunks

½ pointed green or small Savoy cabbage, shredded

2 tbsp olive oil

1 large onion, finely chopped

3 garlic cloves, finely chopped

1 red chilli, finely chopped

½ tsp ground turmeric

1 tsp mustard seeds

100g (3½oz) frozen peas, defrosted or any other cooked greens, finely chopped

100g (3½oz) frozen sweetcorn, defrosted

a few sprigs of any fresh herbs, finely chopped

75g (3oz) Cheddar cheese or similar, grated (optional)

15g (½oz) butter

salt and black pepper

First, cook the potatoes and cabbage. Put the potatoes in a steamer over simmering water and cook until tender – around 10 minutes. To cook the cabbage, either add to the potatoes after they have been cooking for 6 to 7 minutes to steam alongside them or blanch in a little water for a couple of minutes – you want the texture to be quite firm.

Heat half the oil in a frying pan and add the onion. Sauté over a medium-high heat so it takes on some colour as it softens, then add the garlic, chilli, turmeric and mustard seeds. Sauté for another couple of minutes.

Put the potatoes in a bowl and roughly break up, crushed, not mashed. Stir in the cabbage, peas, sweetcorn, onion mixture, herbs and cheese, if using. Season generously with salt and pepper.

Heat the remaining oil and the butter in a large frying pan. Add the bubble-and-squeak mixture and press down evenly across the base of the pan. Cook over a medium-high heat for 5 minutes until it has browned on the underside, then stir. Press down again and cook for another 2 to 3 minutes. Do this a couple more times until the bubble and squeak is flecked with lovely crisp, caramelized brown bits.

Serve while hot, perhaps with a couple of fried or poached eggs.

VARIATION: Chill the mixture for an hour then shape into patties, dust with flour and fry until browned on each side. Or, brush with oil and bake in a 200°C (180°C fan)/gas 6 oven for 20 minutes.

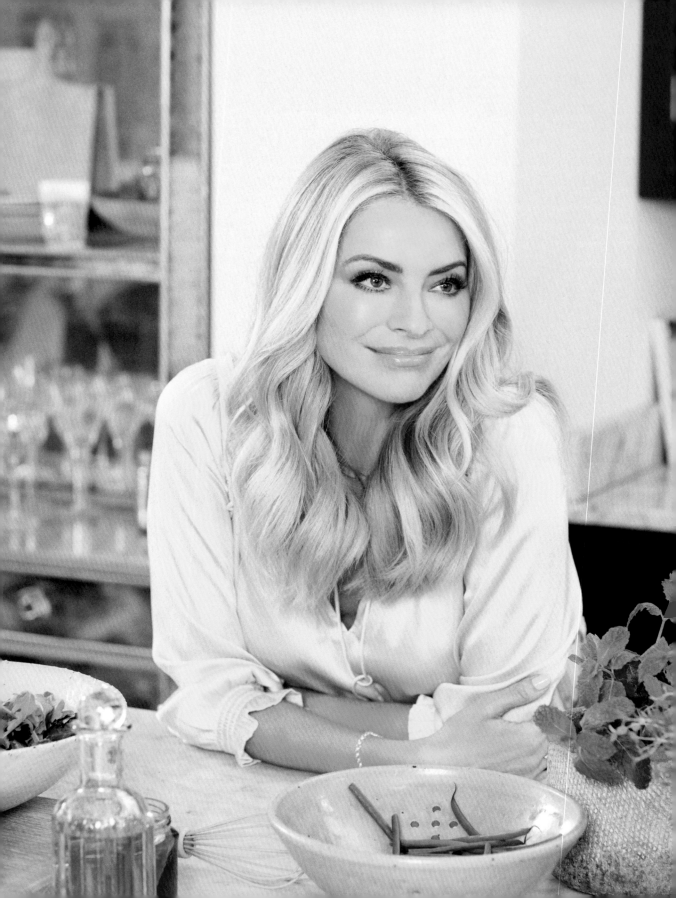

LIGHT BITES
+ SNACKS

Boost your gut microbiome

Pumpkin + Ginger Super-you Soup

PREP 20 MINS
COOK 45 MINS
SERVES 4

2 tbsp oil (olive or coconut)

1 large onion, finely chopped

1 large carrot, peeled and diced

2 celery sticks, diced

1 pumpkin or squash (around 750g/1lb 10oz), peeled and diced

20g (¾oz) root ginger, peeled and grated

4 garlic cloves, crushed

a small bunch of coriander, finely chopped

200g (7oz) tomatoes, chopped (tinned is fine)

1.2 litres (2 pints) vegetable stock

FOR THE SPICE MIX

1 tsp ground turmeric

½ tsp ground coriander

½ tsp ground cardamom

½ tsp ground cumin

½ tsp ground allspice

salt and black pepper

TO GARNISH

1 tbsp olive oil

3 tbsp pumpkin seeds

½ tsp sugar or honey

This simple wholesome soup is fantastically tasty and becomes superhero worthy with the addition of that all-important spice mix and some gut-friendly fresh ginger and garlic. I usually make double batches and freeze some for another day. If you prefer, you can use a bought spice mix, such as baharat, instead of the individual spices.

First, mix the spices together with plenty of black pepper and a generous pinch of salt.

Heat the oil in a large saucepan. Add the onion, carrot, celery and pumpkin or squash and sauté over a medium-low heat until the onion is translucent and the pumpkin is looking soft around the edges.

Add the ginger, garlic and all but ½ teaspoon of the spice mix and continue to cook for a further 2 minutes. Reserve 2 tablespoons of coriander leaves for garnish, then add the rest to the vegetables along with the tomatoes and stock. Season with salt and pepper.

Bring to the boil, then turn down to a simmer and cover. Simmer until all the vegetables are tender – around 20 to 25 minutes.

Blitz until smooth, then reheat.

To make the garnish, heat the oil in a small frying pan and add the pumpkin seeds. Stir in the remaining spice mix, sugar or honey and another pinch of salt and stir until the pumpkin seeds are toasted and smell very aromatic and sweet.

Serve the soup garnished with the pumpkin seeds and reserved coriander.

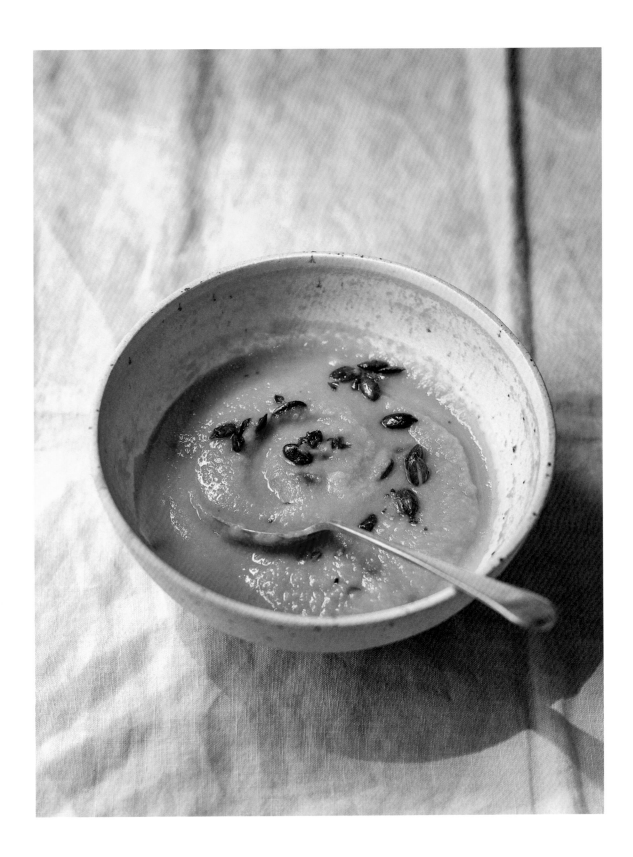

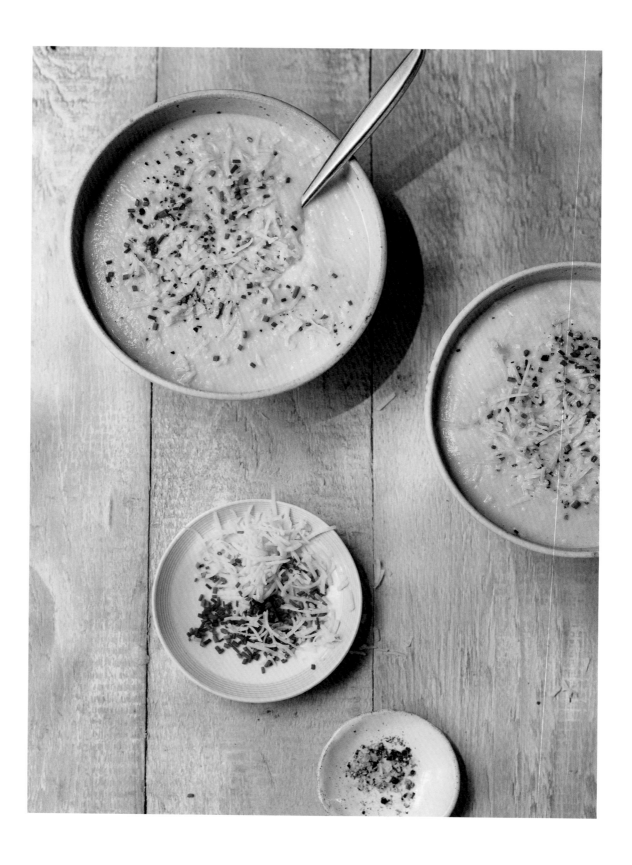

Comforting Cauliflower Cheese Soup

I promise you simply can't go wrong with this warming, people-pleaser of a dish. This soup has a very firm place in my heart since it was literally the first meal I made for our eldest daughter Phoebe when weaning her onto solids. She's eighteen now and she still loves it (admittedly as a more grown-up version) to this day! Cauliflower is a good high-fibre vegetable, rich in nutrients, and I like to add a tin of beans to boost the protein content.

Heat the olive oil and butter in a saucepan and add the onion, celery and cauliflower. Sauté on a medium-high heat for a few minutes until just starting to brown around the edges. Add the garlic and cook for a further 2 minutes, then stir in the mustard.

Add the drained beans and vegetable stock and season with salt and pepper. Bring to the boil, then turn down the heat and leave to simmer until the vegetables are perfectly tender – around 20 minutes.

Blend until smooth, then stir in the milk and cheese. Heat very gently until the cheese has melted into the soup. Serve with any of the garnishes.

PREP 15 MINS
COOK 30 MINS
SERVES 4

1 tbsp olive oil
15g (½oz) butter
1 onion, finely chopped
2 celery sticks, finely chopped
400g (14oz) cauliflower, roughly chopped
2 garlic cloves, finely chopped
2 tsp Dijon mustard
1 × 400g (14oz) tin of cannellini beans
750ml (1¼ pints) vegetable stock
100ml (3½fl oz) milk
100g (3½oz) Cheddar cheese or similar, grated
salt and black pepper

TO GARNISH (OPTIONAL)
25g (1oz) Chedddar cheese or similar, grated
a few snips of chives

Super Crunchy Superfoods Salad

PREP 15 MINS, PLUS STANDING
SERVES 4

FOR THE SALAD

½ large pointed green or red
   cabbage (about 500g/1lb
   2oz), finely shredded

1 large carrot, cut into
   matchsticks or coarsely grated

1 red onion, finely sliced

1 large beetroot, cut into
   matchsticks or coarsely grated

1 tsp salt

2 eating apples, cored and
   diced (preferably unpeeled)

100g (3½oz) baby leaf spinach
   or rocket

100g (3½oz) cooked puy lentils

a handful of mint, coriander and
   parsley, finely chopped

50g (1¾oz) pumpkin seeds

25g (1oz) flaked almonds

FOR THE DRESSING

150g (5½oz) thick live yoghurt
   or kefir

2 tbsp olive or pumpkin oil

1 tbsp raw apple cider vinegar

½ tsp honey

½ tsp wholegrain mustard

salt and black pepper

Kefir or live yoghurt and some apple cider vinegar make this a very gut-friendly salad, and you could also add some sauerkraut if you like. I prefer to keep this vegetarian, but the rest of the family sometimes like to add some smoked mackerel or smoked ham or turkey.

Remember the old saying 'an apple a day keeps the doctor away'? Well, there's a good reason for it. Apples are like toothbrushes for the digestive system. They are rich in a fibre called pectin, which also helps remove toxins from the stomach lining.

First, prepare the cabbage, carrot, onion and beetroot and put them in a large colander. Sprinkle with the salt and toss lightly to combine. Massage the veg gently with your hands – you should see little drops of water start to appear on them. Cover and leave to stand over a bowl for at least half an hour – this helps draw liquid out of the vegetables so they will stay crisp once dressed and also makes the onion a bit less fierce. Gently squeeze the vegetables before transferring them to a bowl.

Whisk all the dressing ingredients together and season with salt and pepper. Add the dressing to the salted vegetables and toss well.

You can serve the salad like this as a coleslaw or leave it in the fridge until you're ready to eat, then add the apple, spinach or rocket leaves and lentils and toss well. Garnish with the herbs, pumpkin seeds and almonds and serve.

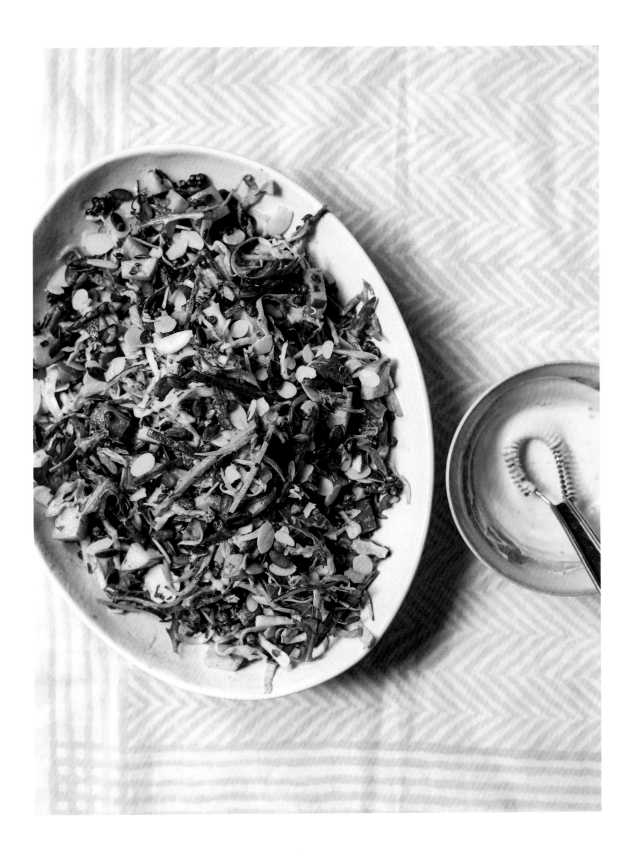

Summer in a Salad

PREP 10 MINS
COOK 3–4 MINS
SERVES 4

300g (10½oz) fine green beans, trimmed and cut into strips
400g (14oz) skinned and diced watermelon
½ cucumber, diced
150g (5½oz) mixed salad leaves
200g (7oz) feta, diced
75g (3oz) pecans, roughly chopped
25g (1oz) sunflower seeds
a few mint leaves

FOR THE SALAD DRESSING
4 tbsp olive oil
2 tbsp raw apple cider vinegar
2 tsp honey
1 red chilli, deseeded and finely chopped
1 garlic clove, halved
salt and black pepper

You couldn't ever accuse me of being a salad-dodger. I love them and I enjoy the challenge of whipping up new summery salads to tempt my girls. Here, the sweet, refreshing watermelon is a wonderful counterpart to the delicate, creamy sharpness of the feta cheese. The crunchy pecans and sunflower seeds add some lovely texture and are great for the gut too, as is the dressing, which is extra gut-friendly thanks to the olive oil, raw apple cider vinegar and garlic.

First, make the salad dressing. Put all the ingredients in a bowl and season with salt and pepper. Whisk, then leave to stand until ready to serve.

Bring a saucepan of water to the boil and add the beans. Cook for 3 to 4 minutes until al dente – they should be a bright green. Drain and refresh under cold water.

Assemble the salad. Gently toss the beans, watermelon, cucumber and salad leaves together. Remove the garlic from the dressing (it will give a hint of flavour, which is all you need here) and drizzle some of it over the salad. Toss again, then top with the feta, pecans and sunflower seeds. Drizzle over a little more dressing. Garnish with a few mint leaves and serve.

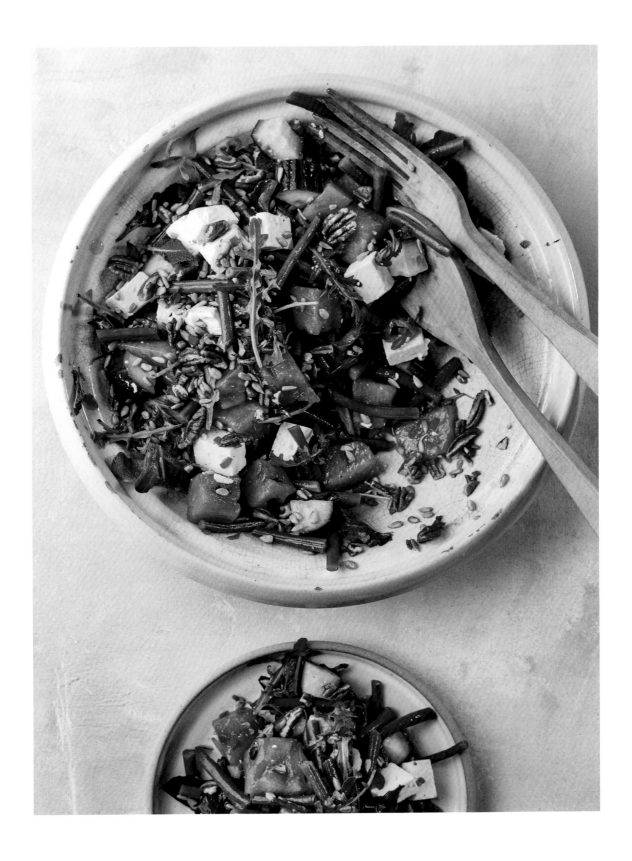

Eat the Rainbow Salad

PREP 20 MINS, PLUS SOAKING
SERVES 4

FOR THE SALAD

½ red onion, finely sliced

3 oranges

150g (5½oz) mixed salad leaves
   or 1 large butterhead lettuce

2 avocados, peeled and diced

juice of ½ lime

3 cooked beetroot, diced

50g (1¾oz) flaked almonds

1 tsp sesame seeds

a few mint or coriander leaves

FOR THE DRESSING

15g (½oz) white miso

1 tsp sesame oil

1 tsp rice wine vinegar or raw
   apple cider vinegar

1 tsp soy sauce

10g (¼oz) root ginger, grated

1 tsp honey (optional)

It may not be everyone's idea of fun (some get positively grumpy), but I absolutely LOVE mixing fruit and vegetables in a salad. It's the sweet and savoury that gets me every time – the unexpected juxtaposition of flavours. Not tried oranges in a salad before? You can thank me afterwards! This salad is packed with plant nutrients and the miso, ginger and orange dressing pops with flavour and complements it perfectly.

First, soak the red onion in salted water for half an hour.

Meanwhile, prepare the oranges. Using a sharp knife, slice a round from the top and bottom of each one, then place on a chopping board and cut away the skin and outer membrane, following the contour of the orange. Hold each orange over a bowl to catch any juice, then trim off any remaining membrane and pith. Take each piece of cut-off peel and squeeze to extract any juice from any flesh, then discard. Add the lime juice. Slice the oranges. You should find you end up with 3 to 4 tablespoons of orange juice, as well as the orange slices.

Add the miso, sesame oil, vinegar, soy sauce and ginger to the orange juice and mix thoroughly. Taste and add a little honey if you feel it needs it – this very much depends on how sweet your orange juice is.

Arrange the salad leaves in a bowl, pour over half the dressing and toss. Add the orange, avocado, beetroot and drained red onion and drizzle over more of the dressing. Garnish with the nuts, seeds and herbs. Serve immediately.

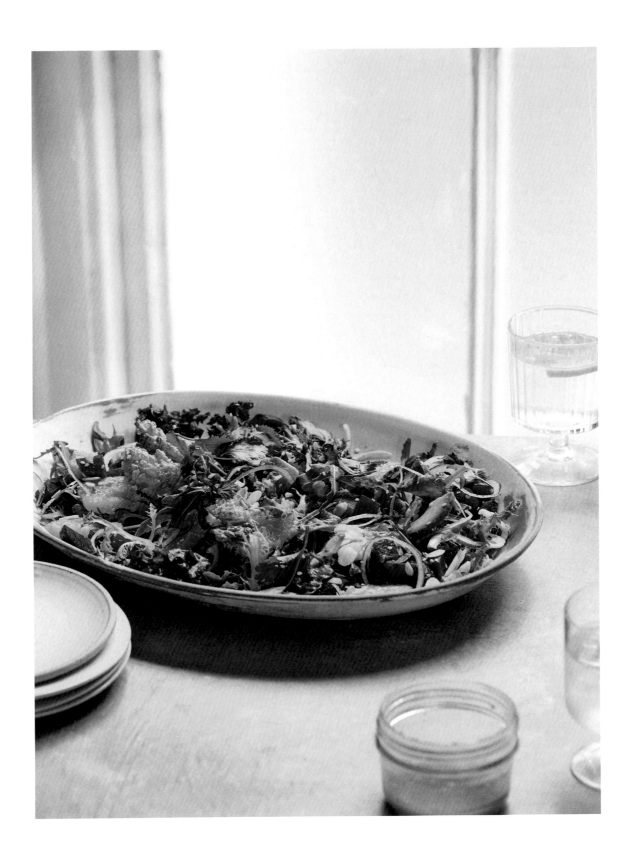

Gently Fermented Coleslaw

PREP 15 MINS, PLUS STANDING
SERVES 4

½ pointed green cabbage
   (around 300g/10½oz),
   shredded
½ red cabbage, shredded
1 large carrot, julienned
50g (1¾oz) radishes, julienned
½ red pepper, very finely sliced
1 small onion, finely chopped
1 eating apple, cored and
   grated (unpeeled)
1 tsp salt
a squeeze of lemon or lime juice
1 tsp raw apple cider vinegar
1 tsp caster sugar or honey
1 tsp ground turmeric
10g (¼oz) root ginger, grated
1 red chilli, finely chopped
½ tsp each mustard and
   sesame seeds
black pepper

FOR THE DRESSING
75g (3oz) thick live yoghurt
75g (3oz) mayonnaise
1 tsp sesame oil
1 tsp Dijon mustard (optional)
1 tbsp raw apple cider vinegar
salt and black pepper

TO SERVE
any soft herbs, finely chopped

We are coleslaw fanatics at our house and it's the one thing we always have in our fridge – alongside eggs and avocados, of course! We eat the stuff with pretty much everything. There's a little fermentation in the prep of this yummy coleslaw and fermented foods are super-good for your gut. I've suggested a selection of vegetables but feel free to vary as you like, being sure to make it as rainbow a selection as possible so you get a good range of plant nutrients. My advice is to prep and lightly brine the vegetables, then keep them in the fridge ready to dress and finish off the salad when needed.

Put the vegetables and apple into a colander. Sprinkle over the teaspoon of salt, lemon juice, the cider vinegar and sugar or honey. Toss well to coat, scrunching everything with your hands as you do so, then place the colander over a bowl or in the sink and leave to stand for an hour – this will draw some of the liquid out of the vegetables and stop your coleslaw from being soggy. Squeeze lightly, then transfer to a container.

Season with pepper and add all the remaining salad ingredients. Leave in the fridge until you're ready to add the dressing and serve. You can keep the vegetables like this for up to a week and they will improve their flavour during that time – they can also be eaten without the dressing.

Make the dressing by mixing all the ingredients together. Season with salt and pepper. Dress the vegetables just before serving and stir in plenty of freshly chopped herbs.

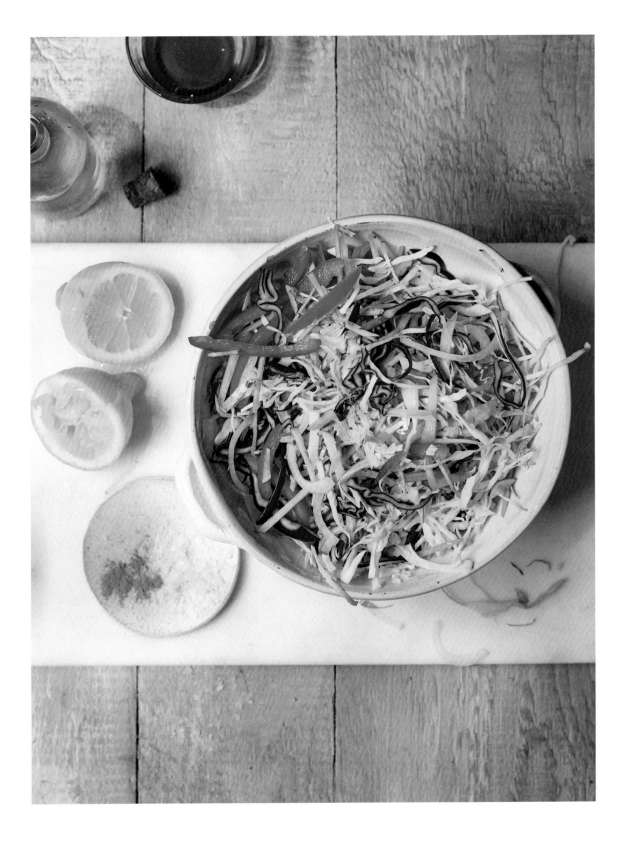

Gorgeously Griddled Aubergine Salad

PREP 15 MINS
COOK UP TO 25 MINS
(DEPENDING ON METHOD
FOR AUBERGINES)
SERVES 4

3 aubergines, cut into 2cm
  (¾ inch) rounds
50ml (1¾fl oz) olive oil
2 tsp dried mixed herbs
seeds from ½ pomegranate
25g (1oz) flaked almonds
a few mint leaves
1–2 tsp za'atar
salt and black pepper

FOR THE DRESSING
a large pinch of saffron
a large pinch of sea salt
1 tbsp tahini
juice of 1 small lemon
200g (7oz) live yoghurt or kefir
1 small garlic clove, crushed
½ tsp honey (optional)

FOR THE GREEN SALAD
100g (3½oz) mixed salad leaves
50g (1¾oz) mixed herbs (mint,
  dill, parsley, coriander, basil)
1 small courgette, very finely
  sliced
1 tbsp olive oil
juice of ½ lemon

I do love the soft, melting texture of griddled aubergines and this salad is the perfect way to enjoy them. Have it as part of a mezze or serve with flatbreads and/or hummus to make a whole meal. The aubergines can be cooked in advance and kept in the fridge for several days until needed if you want to prepare ahead. Just bring them to room temperature before serving. The pomegranate seeds add extra crunch and flavour – and they are rich in fibre and antioxidants too.

To cook the aubergines, you have two options. Brush the aubergine slices with oil and sprinkle with salt and mixed herbs. Then either cook for a few minutes on each side on a large griddle pan or preheat the oven to 200°C (180°C fan)/gas 6, arrange over two to three baking trays and roast for 25 minutes until lightly browned with softened flesh. Remove from the oven and leave to cool to room temperature.

To make the dressing, crush the saffron with a large pinch of sea salt. Mix the tahini with the lemon juice to loosen up the tahini until it is smooth and lump-free, then stir in the saffron, yoghurt and garlic. Taste and add the honey if you would like it slightly sweetened.

To assemble, put the salad leaves, herbs and courgette in a bowl. Season with salt and pepper and drizzle over the olive oil and lemon juice. Spread over a large platter. Arrange the aubergine slices over the top, then garnish with the pomegranate seeds, almonds, mint leaves and za'atar. Drizzle over a small amount of the dressing before serving and leave the rest in a bowl to be added individually at the table.

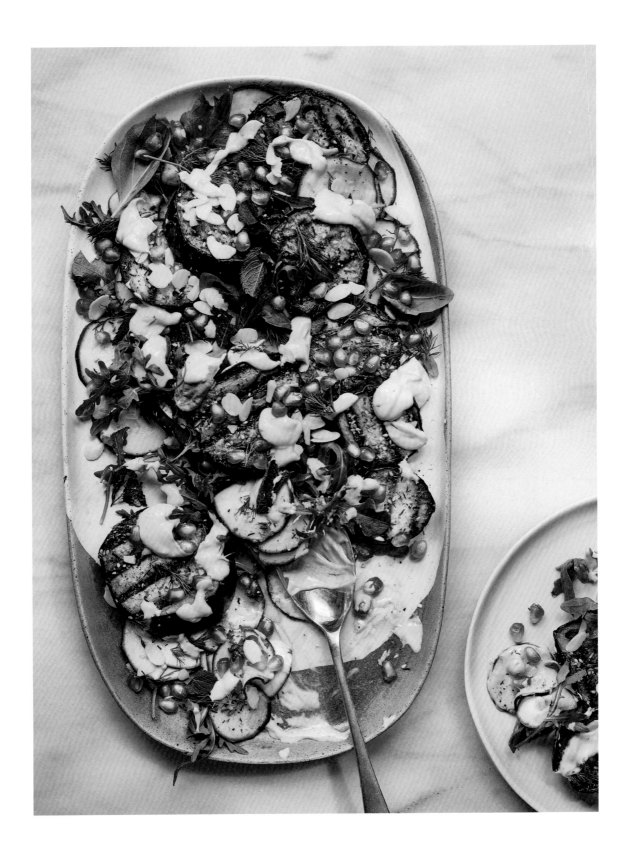

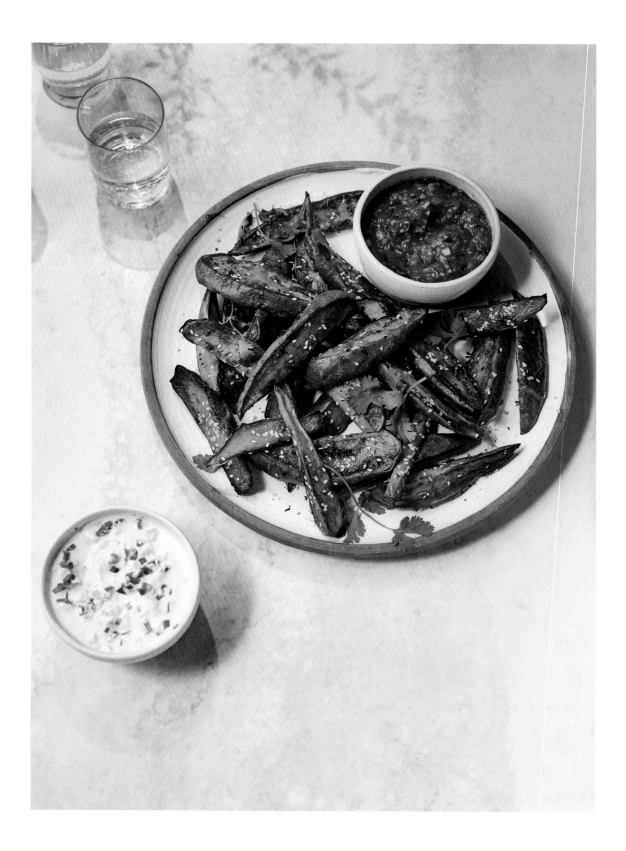

V

Comfort food done healthily is pretty much my cooking mantra. These yummy sweet potato wedges are ideal for boosting your fibre intake – especially with the skins on as here. They work well on their own or as a side dish with your favourite protein. I've made the soy and rosemary optional, but they add a lovely flavour and the sesame seeds provide extra protein. The tomato salsa is easy to make and can be cooked beside the potato wedges.

To make the wedges, preheat the oven to 200°C (180°C fan)/gas 6.

Wash and dry the sweet potatoes, then cut in half crossways and cut each half into wedges.

Toss in the soy sauce, if using, followed by the olive oil. Arrange over a large baking tray, season with salt and pepper, then sprinkle with the rosemary and/or sesame seeds (again, if using). Roast in the oven for 25 to 30 minutes until well browned and tender inside.

To make the tomato salsa put the tomatoes, garlic cloves and jalapeños on a baking tray. Sprinkle the tomatoes with salt, then roast in the oven for around 20 minutes. Leave to cool.

While the tomatoes are roasting, toss the onion in the lime zest and juice and salt. Leave to stand for half an hour. Stir the onion mixture through the processed tomatoes and add the olive oil, vinegar, turmeric and coriander. Taste for seasoning and add more salt, pepper and a pinch of sugar or drizzle of honey, if necessary.

Squeeze the flesh from the garlic cloves and put in a food processor with the tomatoes and jalapeños – you can peel first if you prefer, but they are better for you with the skin on. Pulse until broken down but still fairly chunky.

To make the yoghurt dip, put all the ingredients in a bowl and season with salt and pepper. Mix thoroughly.

Serve the sweet potato wedges with the roast tomato salsa and yoghurt dip.

Sweet Potato Wedges with Fiery Tomato Salsa

PREP 20 MINS
COOK 30 MINS
SERVES 4

4 medium sweet potatoes
1 tbsp soy sauce (optional)
2 tbsp olive oil
1 tsp dried rosemary/finely chopped needles (optional)
1 tsp sesame seeds (optional)
salt and black pepper

FOR THE ROAST TOMATO SALSA
300g (10½oz) cherry tomatoes
4 garlic cloves, unpeeled
2 jalapeños or similar, halved and deseeded
½ red onion, finely chopped
zest and juice of 1 lime
¼ teaspoon salt
1 tbsp olive oil
1 tsp sherry or red wine vinegar
a pinch of ground turmeric
2 sprigs of coriander, chopped
a pinch of sugar or drizzle of honey

FOR THE YOGHURT DIP
250g (9oz) live yoghurt/kefir
50g (1¾oz) cheese, grated
2 spring onions or chives, chopped
¼ tsp honey
1 tsp white wine vinegar

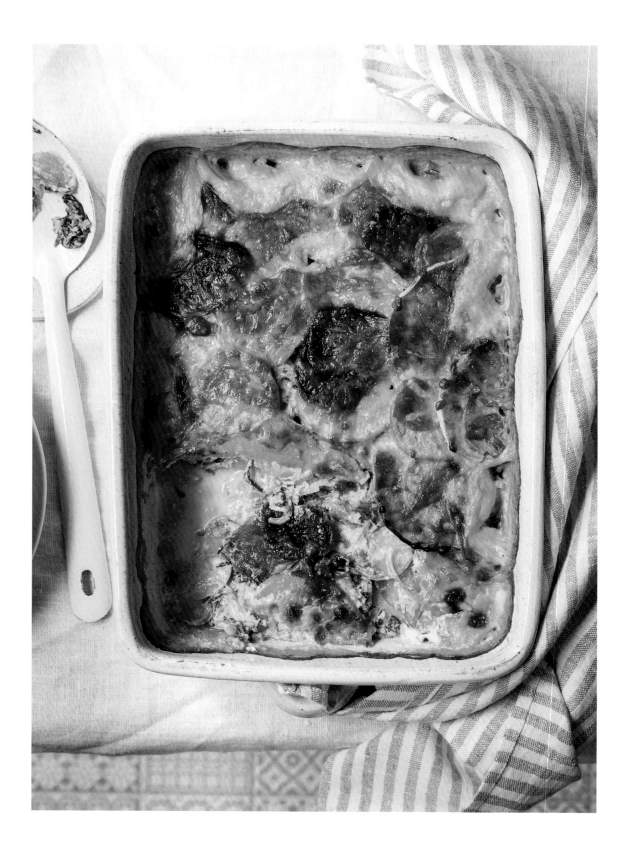

Deeply Delicious Dauphinoise

A classic dauphinoise is made with just potatoes, but try mixing in some other root veg as well, such as carrot, parsnip, sweet potato, celeriac or beetroot, to ramp up the flavour and nutrient content. This forms the basis of a wonderfully hearty supper and is a regular request from my family. The double cream may seem a tad decadent, but it truly is a worthwhile addition. The greens elevate the dish, bringing colour and a welcome nutritional punch too.

PREP 20 MINS
COOK 1 HOUR 10 MINS
SERVES 4

15g (½oz) butter
1 garlic clove, halved
1kg (2lb 4oz) mix of potatoes, other root vegetables and/or squashes
150g (5½oz) frozen spinach, defrosted or 200g (7oz) chard or kale (optional)
1 leek, finely sliced
leaves from a large sprig of thyme or 2 tsp dried mixed herbs
300ml (10½fl oz) double cream
200ml (7fl oz) whole milk
a grating of nutmeg
100g (3½oz) Cheddar cheese or similar, grated
salt and black pepper

Preheat your oven to 180°C (160°C fan)/gas 4.

Take an oven dish and rub it with butter, followed by the cut halves of garlic.

Prepare your vegetables. Peel any that need peeling (potatoes and carrots are best left unpeeled) and slice as thinly as you can, preferably with a mandolin.

If using chard or kale, separate the leaves from the stems and finely chop both. Blanch in boiling water for 2 minutes, then drain thoroughly and squeeze out any excess water. If using spinach, again, make sure you squeeze out any excess water, then finely chop.

Finely chop the garlic halves.

Layer up the vegetables in your oven dish, starting and finishing with the root vegetables or squash and making sure you have two layers of greens between the root vegetables, if using. Sprinkle the leek, garlic and herbs throughout the layers, remembering to season with salt and pepper as you assemble.

Mix the double cream and milk together and pour over the vegetables. Press them down into the liquid – it should almost reach the top of the dish. Cover with foil and bake for 30 to 40 minutes (40 minutes if using carrot and/or beetroot, 30 for everything else).

Remove the foil and press down the vegetables again. Grate over a little nutmeg, then top with the cheese. Bake in the oven for a further 30 minutes until the top is well browned and bubbling and the vegetables are tender.

Happy Place Chicken Soup

PREP 20 MINS
COOK ABOUT 40 MINS
SERVES 4

1 tbsp olive oil

15g (½oz) butter

1 onion, diced

3 celery sticks, diced

2 carrots, diced

3 garlic cloves, finely chopped

a large sprig of thyme

2 bay leaves

300g (10½oz) potatoes, sliced

3 leeks, sliced into 2cm
  (¾ inch) rounds

1 litre (1¾ pints) well-flavoured
  chicken stock

150g (5½oz) cavolo nero, kale
  or chard, shredded

250g (9oz) cooked chicken,
  diced or pulled

150g (5½oz) frozen peas,
  defrosted

salt and black pepper

TO SERVE (OPTIONAL)
freshly grated Parmesan

I'm not sure there's anything more comforting or satisfying than a good, hearty chicken soup. This one really is good for the soul and ideal for lunch on a cold winter day. I usually use cooked chicken but if you prefer to use raw, increase the quantity to about 400g (14oz), cook it right at the start, and then proceed with the rest of the recipe.

Heat the oil and butter in a large saucepan. Add the onion, celery and carrot and sauté over a medium heat until they are starting to take on some colour and softening around the edges.

Add the garlic, herbs, potato and leek. Stir so everything is coated in the oil and butter, then pour in the stock. Season with salt and pepper. Bring to the boil, then turn down the heat and partially cover. Simmer for 15 minutes.

Add the cavolo nero, kale or chard and continue to simmer until all the vegetables are tender – this will take another 10 to 15 minutes. Add the chicken and peas and heat through for a few more minutes.

Taste for seasoning. Remove the thyme sprig and bay leaves before serving with the Parmesan, if using.

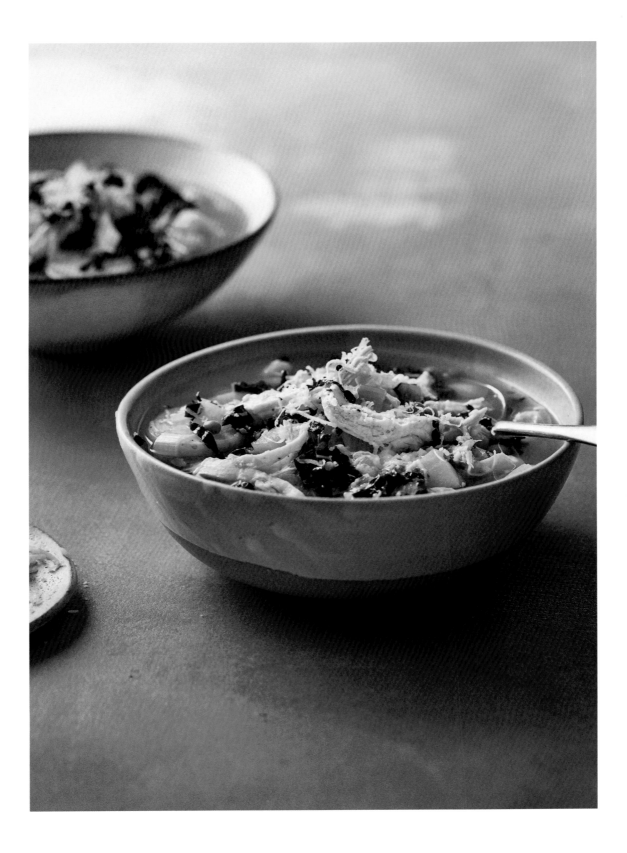

Perfect Marriage Salad

PREP 15 MINS
COOK ABOUT 20 MINS
SERVES 4

350g (12oz) salad or new
  potatoes, unpeeled
350g (12oz) cauliflower florets
1 tbsp olive oil
¼ tsp each nigella, mustard and
  cumin seeds
1 small red onion, finely sliced
150g (5½oz) mixed salad leaves
1 mango, peeled and diced
salt

FOR THE DRESSING
a small bunch of coriander,
  roughly chopped
juice of 1 small lemon
3 tbsp olive oil
¼ tsp each ground turmeric,
  cinnamon and cayenne
  powder
½ tsp honey

TO GARNISH
a few mint leaves
a few coriander leaves
1–2 chillies, finely sliced
  (optional)

'Potato with mango?' I hear you cry … but stick with me and I guarantee you'll be glad you did. Along with the pairing of new potatoes and cauliflower, mango is a wildcard ingredient that marries perfectly with the vegetables. I like the tang and crunch of the raw red onion, but I prefer to soak it first to reduce any bitterness. I've added small amounts of spice, but this doesn't make the salad fiery – just full of flavour.

First, cook the potatoes and cauliflower. Slice the potatoes into 1cm (½ inch) rounds and put in a large saucepan. Cover with water and add ½ teaspoon salt. Bring to the boil and keep boiling, partially covered, for 5 minutes. Add the cauliflower, return to the boil and simmer until the cauliflower is just tender – you want it slightly al dente. Drain the vegetables and run under cold water to cool.

Heat the olive oil in a small frying pan. When hot, add the seeds. Shake the pan a couple of times until the seeds start to pop, then remove from the heat. Pour over the potatoes and cauliflower and toss to coat.

While the vegetables are cooking, put the red onion in a small bowl and sprinkle over salt. Cover with water and leave to stand. Strain just before you assemble the salad.

To make the dressing, put all the ingredients into a small food processor with a generous pinch of salt and blend until you have a bright green dressing. Transfer to a bowl and rinse the processor out with 2 tablespoons water. Add this to the dressing.

To assemble, divide the salad leaves among four bowls. Add the potato, cauliflower, drained onion and mango. Add a tablespoon of the dressing to each bowl and toss lightly. Garnish with the herbs and chilli, if using, and serve immediately.

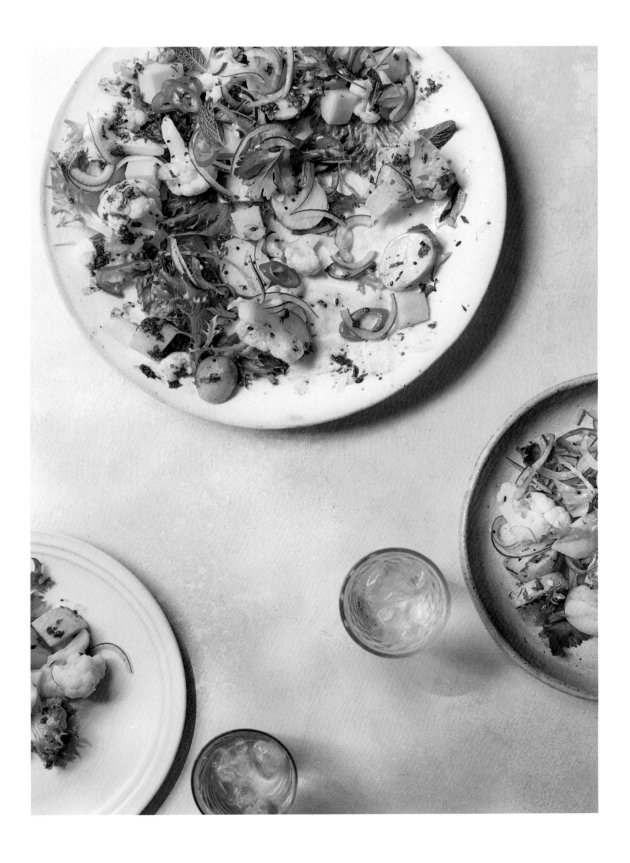

Tantalizing Toast Toppers

Show me a person who doesn't crave the comfort of toast on occasion. My toppings are scrumptious and nutritious and will keep you satisfied all the way till dinner time. I know it's awfully British but a sandwich in any incarnation – particularly one with a healthy twist – is, and always has been, my go-to for lunch. Each of these recipes is enough to top four large slices of sourdough or seeded boule. Pictured overleaf.

Open Tuna Melt

PREP 10 MINS, PLUS MARINATING
COOK ABOUT 5 MINS

½ red onion, finely chopped
juice of ½ lime
1 celery stick, finely chopped
½ red pepper, finely chopped
1 × 160g (5½oz) tin of tuna, drained
1 tbsp capers, chopped
a few coriander or basil leaves, finely chopped
2 tbsp thick live yoghurt, kefir or mayonnaise
4 large slices of sourdough/seeded boule
butter (optional)
½ cucumber, thinly sliced
100g (3½oz) Cheddar cheese or similar, grated
salt and black pepper

Preheat your grill to a medium-high setting.

Toss the red onion in the lime juice with a large pinch of salt. Leave for 20 minutes, then mix with the celery, red pepper, tuna, capers and herbs.

Mix thoroughly, then stir through the yoghurt, kefir or mayonnaise. Taste and adjust the seasoning as necessary.

Lightly toast the bread, then butter if you like. Add the cucumber, followed by the tuna mix, then the grated cheese. Put under the grill, turning around once, until the cheese has melted. Serve immediately.

Roast Cherry Tomatoes

PREP 5 MINS   **COOK** ABOUT 15 MINS

250g (9oz) cherry tomatoes, halved
2 tbsp olive oil
a small handful of basil leaves, finely chopped
4 large slices of sourdough/seeded boule
butter (optional)
100g (3½oz) log goat's cheese, ricotta or curd (optional)
1 tsp balsamic vinegar
sea salt

Preheat your oven to 200°C (180°C fan)/gas 6.

Toss the cherry tomatoes with half the olive oil and arrange, cut-side up, in an oven dish or roasting tin. Sprinkle with half the basil and some sea salt. Roast in the oven for around 15 minutes until softened.

Lightly toast the bread, then butter if you like, and, if using, spread with the cheese, ricotta or curd. Top with the roasted tomatoes, then whisk the remaining oil with the balsamic vinegar and drizzle it over the top. Garnish with a few of the remaining shredded basil leaves and serve.

Open Turkey BLT

PREP 5 MINS   **COOK** 5 MINS

4 large slices of sourdough/seeded boule
1 large avocado, lightly mashed
4 medium tomatoes, sliced
1 tbsp olive oil
1 tsp lemon juice or sherry vinegar
75g (3oz) rocket or mixed salad leaves,
   roughly chopped
12 slices of turkey bacon, grilled or fried (optional)
salt and black pepper

Lightly toast the bread and divide the mashed avocado onto the slices, spreading evenly. Arrange the tomatoes over the top.

Whisk the olive oil and lemon juice or vinegar together and season with salt and pepper, then add the leaves. Toss to coat, then arrange over the top of the tomatoes. Top with the bacon, if using.

Power-up Mashed Banana with Honey + Lime

PREP 5 MINS   **COOK** 2 MINS

4 large slices of sourdough/seeded boule
4 tbsp nut butter (optional)
4 bananas
zest and juice of ½ lime
4 tsp honey, for drizzling
4 tsp sesame seeds or flaked almonds

Lightly toast the bread and spread with nut butter, if using. Roughly mash the bananas and stir in the lime juice and zest. Divide the banana onto the slices of bread and drizzle with honey. Sprinkle with the sesame seeds or almonds.

Bravo for Beetroot + Hummus

PREP 10 MINS   **COOK** 2 MINS

FOR THE HUMMUS
1 × 400g (14oz) tin of chickpeas
1 tbsp tahini
juice of 1 lemon
1 garlic clove, crushed
a generous pinch of ground turmeric
a generous pinch of ground cumin
2 tbsp olive oil
salt and black pepper

FOR THE TOAST
4 large slices of sourdough/seeded boule
2 tbsp pumpkin seeds
4 cooked beetroot, sliced
1 tbsp olive oil
1 tsp lemon juice
60g (2¼oz) mustard leaves or watercress,
   roughly chopped

Put all but 2 tablespoons of the drained chickpeas in a food processor with the tahini, lemon juice, garlic, spices and plenty of seasoning. Pulse until well broken down, then drizzle in the olive oil and enough water to help it process. Roughly mash the remaining chickpeas and stir in to provide some texture.

Lightly toast the bread, then spread with hummus. Sprinkle with the pumpkin seeds and top with the beetroot slices. Whisk the olive oil and lemon juice together, then add the leaves. Toss to coat, then pile on top of the beetroot.

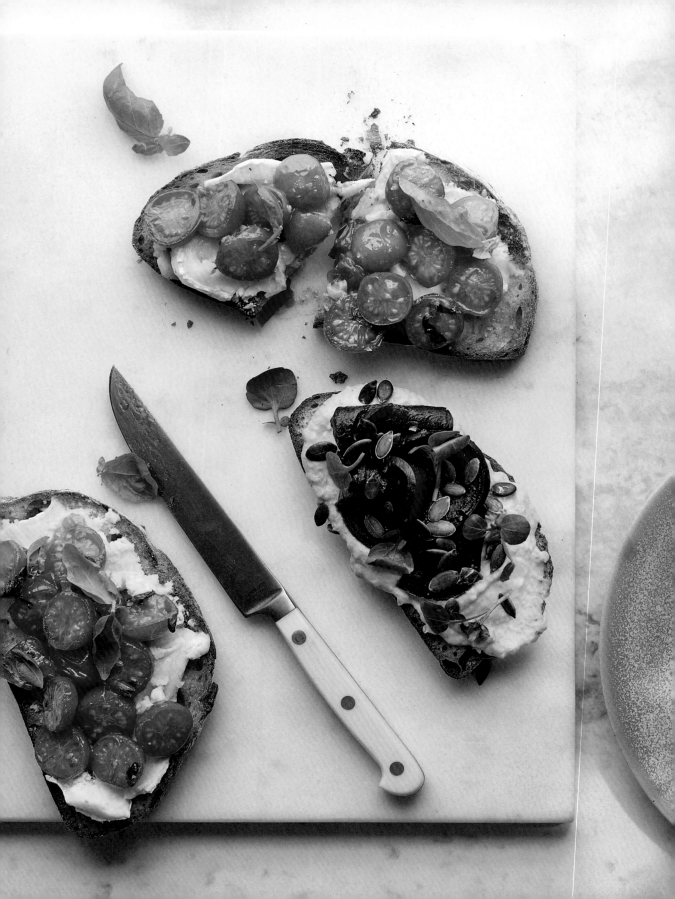

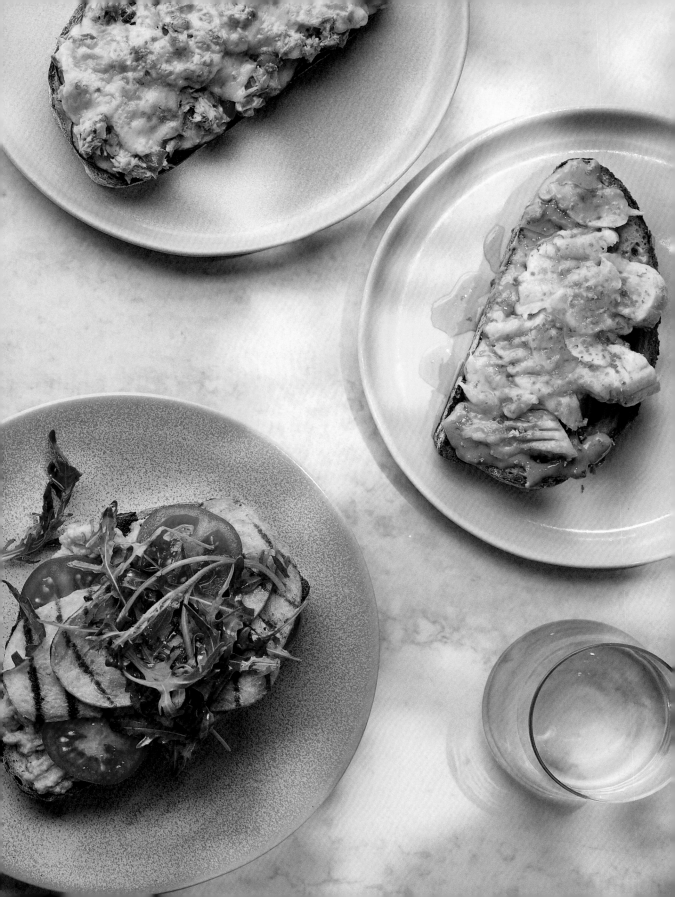

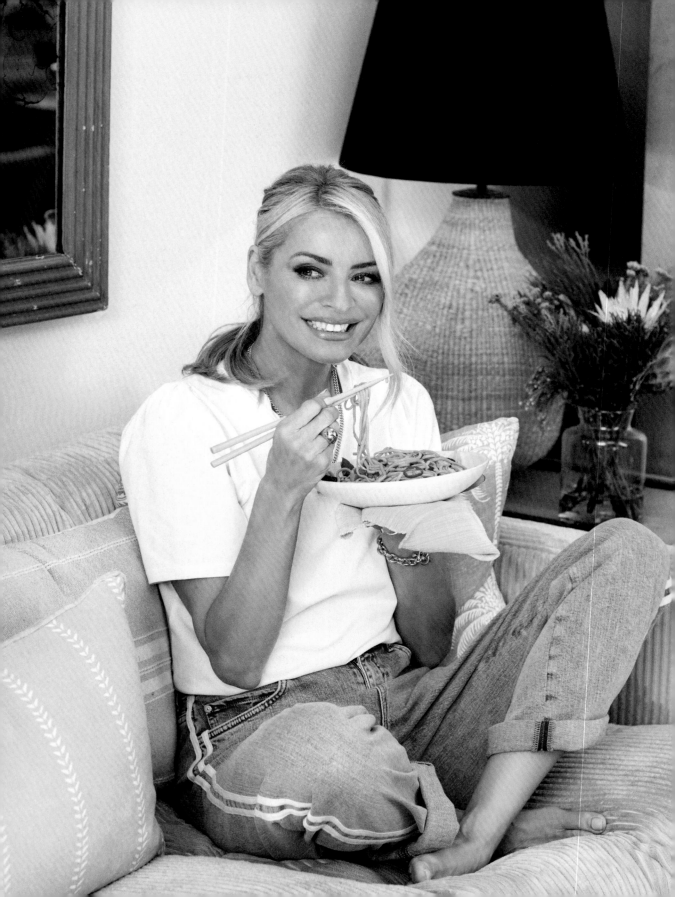

MAIN DISHES

Variety is the spice of life

Potato Pesto Pasta – Perfection

PREP 10 MINS
COOK 10 MINS
SERVES 4

300g (10½oz) pasta
300g (10½oz) salad or new
  potatoes, sliced
1 leek, sliced into 5mm
  (¼ inch) rounds
150g (5½oz) asparagus tips,
  sliced on the diagonal or
  1 courgette, thinly sliced
salt

FOR THE PESTO
50g (1¾oz) basil leaves
½ garlic clove
25g (1oz) pine nuts
25g (1oz) Parmesan or
  vegetarian alternative
a pinch of salt
50ml (1¾fl oz) olive oil

TO FINISH
a squeeze of lemon juice
freshly grated Parmesan

Yummy, quick and economical, this recipe saves on fuel – and washing-up – as the pasta, potatoes and vegetables are all cooked in the same pan. If you think this is some kind of carb coma in the making, think again – gnocchi are pretty much the same combo and they work beautifully. Plenty of fibre content here and if you want extra protein, you could replace the potatoes with some drained cannellini beans. Just add them at the end to warm through.

First, make the pesto. Put the basil leaves, garlic, pine nuts and Parmesan in a food processor with a pinch of salt. Pulse, pushing down regularly, until the basil starts to break down, then drizzle in the oil until you have a bright green, slightly textured paste.

Bring a saucepan of water to the boil and add a heaped teaspoon of salt. Add the pasta and potatoes and cook for around 8 minutes, then add the leek. Continue to cook until the pasta and potatoes are just al dente, then add the asparagus or courgette and cook just for another minute. Drain the pasta and vegetables and return to the saucepan.

Stir in the pesto, then taste. Add a squeeze of lemon if you like, then serve with more Parmesan sprinkled over.

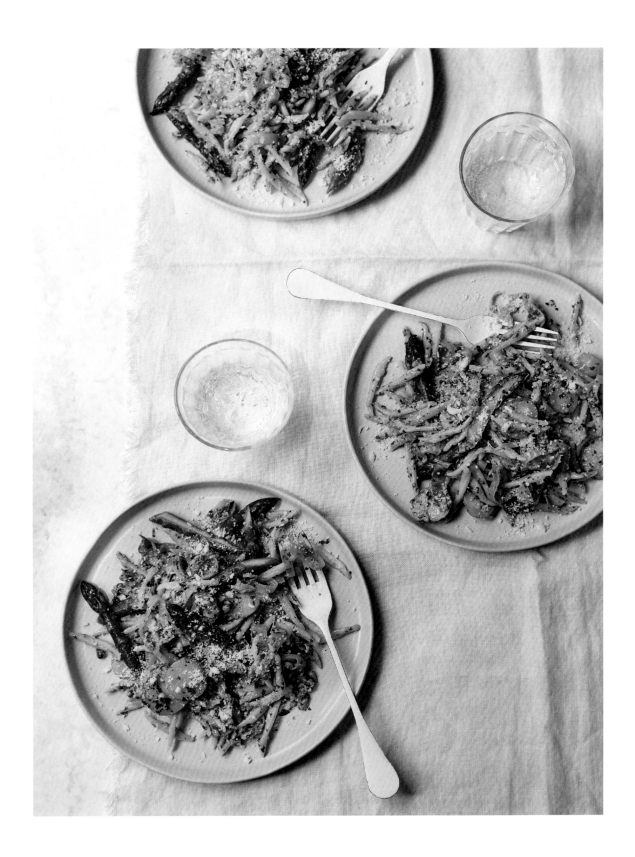

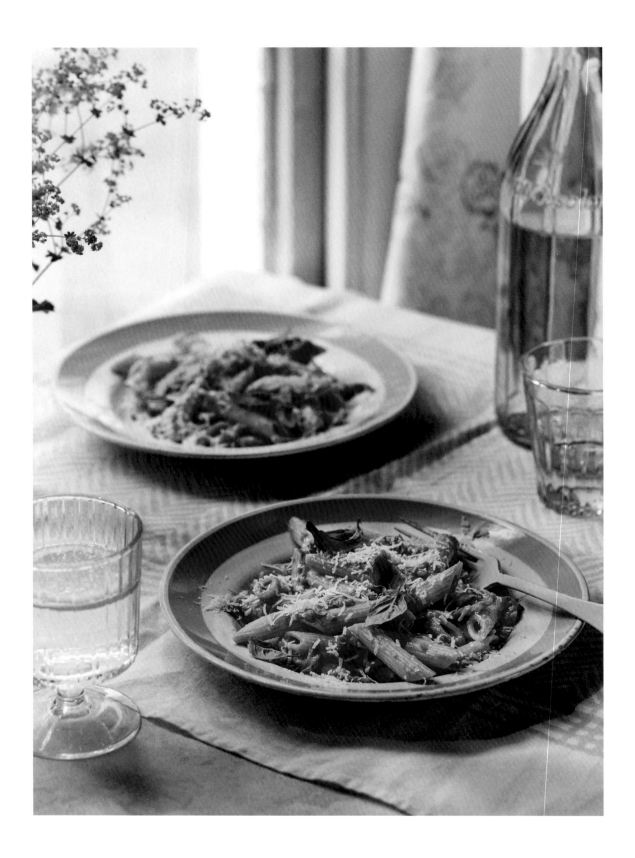

Rollicking Roast Tomato Pasta

This is speedy to make and a popular supper in my house. Baking the tomatoes in the oven makes them BURST with sweet, juicy flavour. My youngest used to refuse tomatoes point-blank until I sneakily popped these oven-baked beauties into her pasta and now there's no going back! It's a healthy dish too, as tomatoes are rich in fibre, vitamin C, lycopene, vitamin K and other nutrients. If you prefer, you can use cream cheese or curds instead of yoghurt.

PREP 10 MINS
COOK 25 MINS
SERVES 4

400g (14oz) cherry tomatoes, halved
4 garlic cloves, unpeeled
1 tsp Italian mixed herbs
2 tbsp olive oil
400g (14oz) penne
½–1 tsp chilli flakes
2 tbsp thick live yoghurt
salt and black pepper

TO SERVE
a few basil leaves
freshly grated Parmesan or vegetarian alternative (optional)

Preheat the oven to 200°C (180°C fan)/gas 6. Put the cherry tomatoes and garlic cloves into a roasting tin or ovenproof dish and sprinkle with the herbs. Season with salt and pepper then drizzle over the olive oil. Roast in the oven for 20 to 25 minutes until the tomatoes have burst and the garlic has softened. Remove from the oven. Squish the flesh from the garlic and discard the skins. Put in a food processor or blender with the tomatoes. Blend very briefly – you don't want to completely break down the tomatoes – then set aside.

While the tomatoes are roasting, bring a large pot of water to the boil and add a heaped teaspoon of salt. Add the penne and cook until al dente – around 12 minutes. Drain and return to the saucepan.

Pour the sauce over the penne and add the chilli flakes and yoghurt. Stir until the sauce looks well combined and creamy.

Divide among four bowls and garnish with a few basil leaves, grated Parmesan and plenty of freshly ground black pepper.

Sizzling Sweet + Sour Stir Fry

PREP 15 MINS
COOK 15 MINS
SERVES 4

FOR THE STIR-FRY

2 tbsp neutral-tasting
   oil
2 large chicken breasts,
   finely sliced
1 large carrot, cut into
   thin batons
1 red pepper, cut into
   strips
175g (6oz) baby corn,
   cut in half diagonally
200g (7oz) asparagus
   tips, cut into 4cm
   (1½ inch) lengths
100g (3½oz) bok choi
   or similar, cut into
   wedges
a bunch of spring
   onions, whites and
   greens separated, cut
   into rounds
3 garlic cloves, finely
   chopped
10g (¼oz) root ginger,
   finely chopped into
   matchsticks
200g (7oz) fresh
   pineapple, diced
1 tsp sesame oil
a few sprigs of
   coriander, finely
   chopped

FOR THE SAUCE

3 tbsp soy sauce
1 tbsp rice wine
   (Shaoxing or mirin)
1 tbsp rice wine vinegar
1 tbsp hot sauce or 1 tsp
   chilli flakes
1 tsp sesame oil
1 tsp honey or kecap
   manis (sweetened soy
   sauce)
50ml (1¾fl oz)
   pineapple juice
salt

TO SERVE

2 packs of cooked
   noodles (around
   550g/1lb 4oz) or 200g
   (7oz) medium egg
   noodles

This is my kids' favourite and I must admit to being extremely partial to it myself. It's sweet, thanks to the pineapple, yet the root ginger and spring onions give it added bite and nutritional value. It's hard to get enough veg for everyone into one wok, so what I do is cook the noodles separately, then just mix them with the chicken and vegetables at the end. If you like, you can substitute some of the noodles with beansprouts and for a vegetarian version, leave out the chicken.

First, whisk all the sauce ingredients together and season with salt.

Cook the noodles according to the packet instructions.

Heat half the oil in a large wok. When the air above the oil starts to shimmer, it will be hot enough. Add the chicken and stir-fry very quickly until the chicken is just cooked through. Remove from the wok.

Add the remaining oil and again, wait for the air to shimmer. Add the carrot, pepper and baby corn and stir-fry for several minutes until the carrot is almost cooked. Add the asparagus tips, bok choi and spring onion whites along with the garlic and ginger. Continue to cook until the vegetables are al dente and the leaves of the bok choi have wilted down.

Return the chicken to the wok and add the pineapple. Pour over the sauce and simmer, stirring constantly, until everything is piping hot. Carefully stir in the noodles and spring onion greens.

Divide among four large plates and sprinkle with sesame oil and coriander.

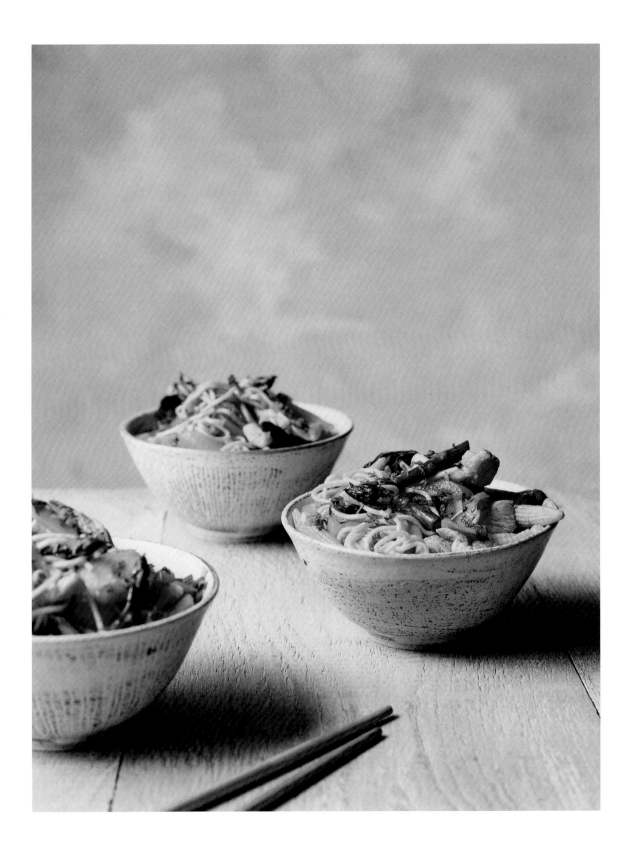

Fill-me-up Funky Frittata

PREP 15 MINS
COOK 40 MINS
SERVES 4

2 medium sweet potatoes, peeled and diced
1 red pepper, diced
1 green pepper (or another red pepper), diced
2 red onions, cut into wedges
1 courgette, diced
2 tbsp olive oil
15g (½oz) butter
1 red chilli, finely chopped
2 garlic cloves, finely chopped
½ tsp ground turmeric
a few sprigs of soft herbs (basil, coriander, mint, tarragon, anything you like), shredded
75g (3oz) frozen peas, defrosted
6 eggs, well beaten
200g (7oz) feta, cubed
salt and black pepper

Great served at brunch or as a main meal, this is quick and easy to prepare. I've absolutely loaded it with vegetables and it should come out beautifully tender but still firm enough to slice. I've suggested my favourite veg, but you can ring the changes and it's a good way to use up any odds and ends in the fridge. You can also use a creamy goat's cheese instead of feta if you prefer.

Preheat your oven to 200°C (180°C fan)/gas 6.

Put the sweet potato, peppers, onion and courgette in a roasting tin and drizzle over half the oil. Season with salt and pepper, then cover with foil and bake for 20 minutes. Remove the foil and check the vegetables are tender, then continue to cook, uncovered, for a further 10 minutes.

Meanwhile, heat the remaining oil and butter in a large non-stick frying pan or well-seasoned skillet. Add the chilli and garlic and sauté for 2–3 minutes just to take away the harsh raw flavour from the garlic. Stir in the turmeric.

Add the roast vegetables, the herbs and the peas and stir to coat in the oil. Season the eggs with salt and pepper, then pour this around the vegetables. Top with the cheese.

Preheat your grill to medium-high. Cook the frittata over a high heat until you can see the underside has set and browned, then transfer to the grill and continue to cook until the eggs are set and have puffed up slightly. The cheese will be soft and creamy.

Leave to stand for a few minutes, then carefully cut into wedges. Good hot or cold.

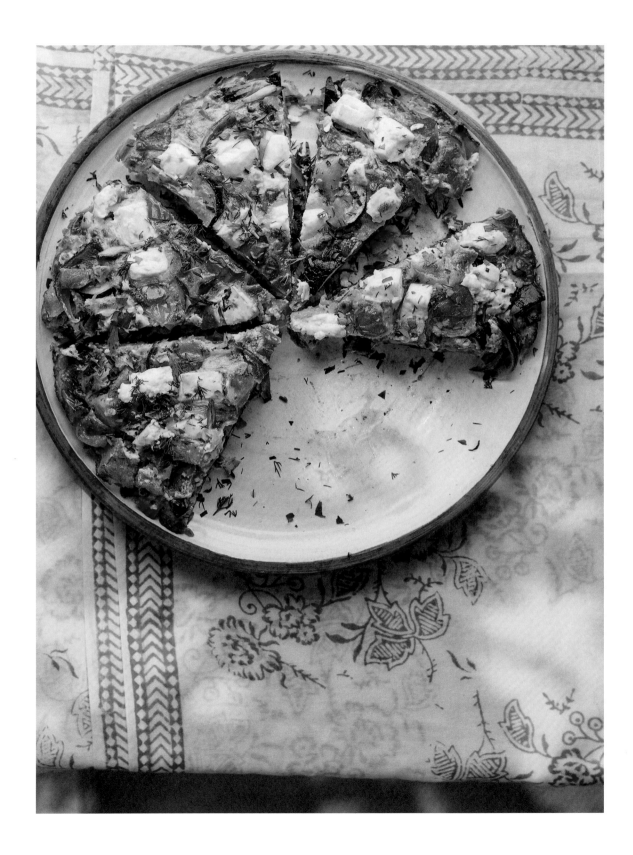

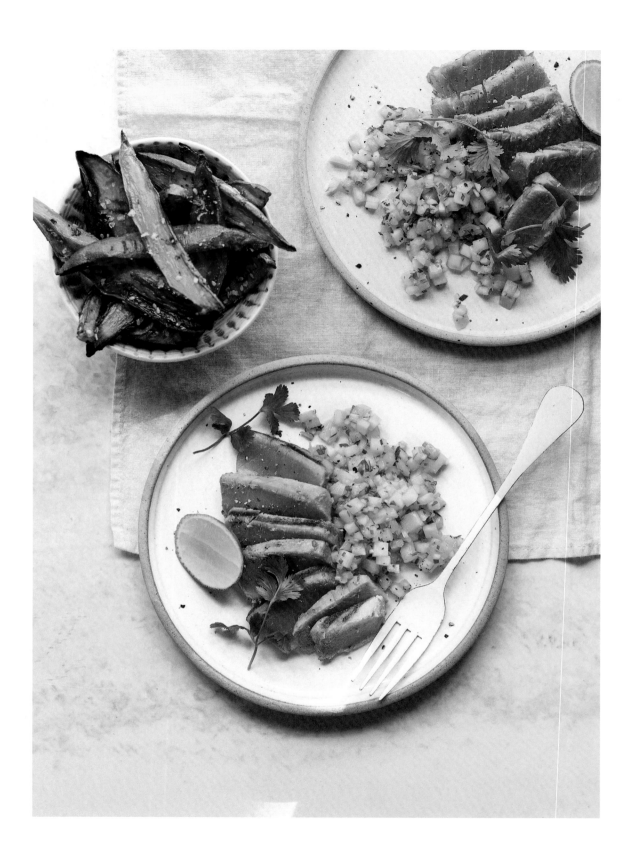

Marinated Tuna with Mango + Pineapple Salsa

Hand on heart, if it were left to me, I'd include pineapple in some incarnation in EVERY dish I serve at home! I can't get enough of the stuff. It drives Claudia nuts when we're sharing a pizza at work, as I have to have some on my half! Makes me giggle every time. Pineapple is even better when paired with mango and works wonderfully well as a salsa for fresh tuna, which is an oily fish, so good for boosting your omega-3 levels. I like to serve this dish with either sweet potato fries from page 83 or sweet potato mash – simply bake sweet potatoes in the oven, scoop out the insides and mash lightly with a fork – and a watercress salad.

First, marinate the tuna. Mix the oil, ginger, garlic, lime zest, soy sauce and hot sauce together. Season the tuna with salt and pepper, then add to the marinade, making sure it is completely coated. Marinate for at least half an hour. If you want to make this in advance, you can leave it in the fridge, but make sure you remove it half an hour before you want to cook it so it can return to room temperature.

To make the salsa, mix everything together and season with salt and pepper.

When you are ready to cook the tuna, heat a griddle pan until it is too hot to hold your hand over. Brush the marinade off the tuna and cook to your liking. For the best (tender) texture, searing for a minute or two on each side until char lines appear, but keeping it still rare in the centre, is ideal. Baste with the marinade as it cooks.

Serve the tuna with the salsa.

PREP 10 MINS, PLUS MARINATING
COOK 5 MINS
SERVES 4

FOR THE TUNA
4 tuna steaks
1 tbsp olive oil
15g (½oz) root ginger, grated
2 garlic cloves, grated
zest of 1 lime
2 tbsp soy sauce
1 tsp hot sauce (preferably smoked)
salt and black pepper

FOR THE SALSA
1 mango, peeled and finely diced
125g (4½oz) pineapple, finely diced
1 small or ½ red onion, finely chopped
1 red chilli, finely diced
1 tsp honey
juice of 1 lime
a few sprigs of coriander, finely chopped

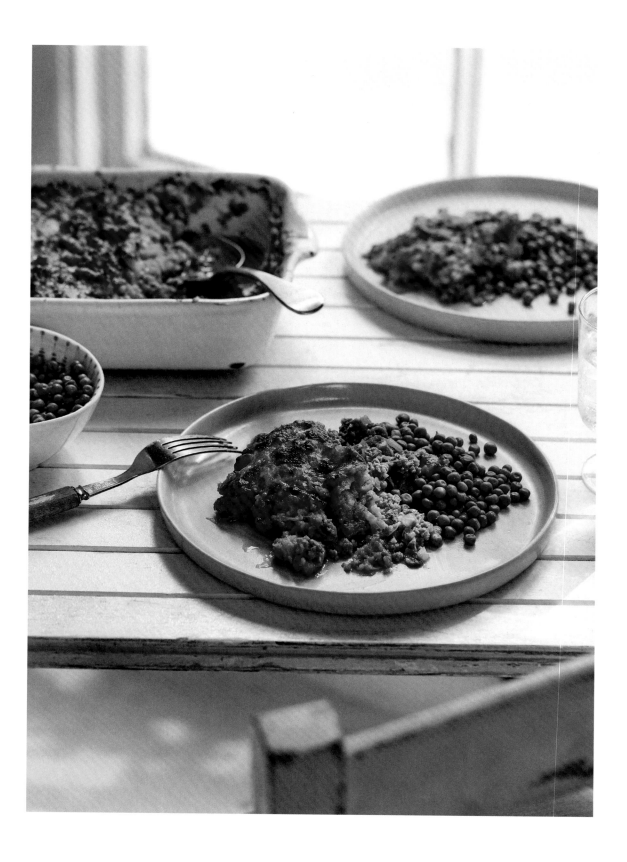

I've not eaten anything that would be herded by a shepherd since I was 16 years old, so I find turkey mince a much more pleasing option for a shepherd's pie than the usual red meat – it's healthier too! I top it with a mash of carrots and swede or pumpkin, which is light and delicious and ups your veg intake. This is a winner, and any leftovers can be warmed up the next day for a no-brainer supper.

Crowd-pleaser Turkey Shepherd's Pie

PREP 25 MINS
COOK ABOUT 1 HOUR
SERVES 4

2 tbsp olive oil
1 onion, finely chopped
2 celery sticks, finely chopped
2 garlic cloves, finely chopped
200g (7oz) white cup
  mushrooms, sliced
2 large leeks, thickly sliced
a few sprigs of tarragon
a few sprigs of thyme
500g (1lb 2oz) turkey mince
2 tbsp tomato purée
100ml (3½fl oz) white wine
150ml (5fl oz) chicken stock
a small bunch of parsley,
  finely chopped
sea salt and black pepper

FOR THE TOPPING
1 large swede or pumpkin
  (about 500g/1lb 2oz), peeled
  and diced
500g (1lb 2oz) carrots, peeled
  and diced
2 tbsp crème fraîche
75g (3oz) Cheddar cheese,
  grated (optional) or 1 tbsp
  butter

First, make the filling. Heat the olive oil in a large pan and add the onion, celery, garlic, mushroom, leek and herbs. Stir to coat everything in the oil, then season with salt and cover the pan. Leave over a very low heat for about 10 minutes, stirring at intervals, until the vegetables are just tender.

Turn up the heat and add the turkey mince, breaking it up with a wooden spoon. Stir until the mince is lightly browned, then stir in the tomato purée, followed by the white wine and stock. Season with salt and pepper, then cover the pan and leave to simmer for 10 minutes. Remove the lid and if it looks like there is a lot of liquid in the mixture, allow it to reduce for a few more minutes. Take the pan off the heat, remove the herb sprigs and stir through the chopped parsley.

While the filling is cooking, make the topping. Put the swede or pumpkin and the carrot in a lidded steamer basket and set over a pan of boiling water. Season with salt and steam for about 15 minutes until tender. Tip the veg into a dry saucepan and leave to steam over a low heat for 5 minutes to help get rid of some of the excess water. Mash thoroughly, then check for seasoning and stir in the crème fraîche.

Preheat the oven to 200°C (180°C fan)/gas 6. Spoon the filling into a large ovenproof dish (about 20 × 30cm/8 × 12 inches), then top with the swede and carrot mash. Sprinkle the grated cheese on top, if using, or dot with butter. Bake in the oven for 25 to 30 minutes until lightly browned.

Cheesy Baked Cod

PREP 20 MINS
COOK 25-30 MINS
SERVES 4

FOR THE CHEESE SAUCE
25g (1oz) butter
25g (1oz) plain flour
400ml (14fl oz) milk
100g (3½oz) Cheddar cheese,
 grated
1 tsp mustard
salt and black pepper

FOR THE COD
4 pieces of cod loin or fillet (or
 similar, haddock, etc.), skinned
30g (1oz) breadcrumbs
2 tbsp capers, chopped
2 tbsp gherkins or pickled
 jalapeños, finely chopped
leaves from 2 large sprigs of
 basil, finely chopped
leaves from 2 sprigs of tarragon,
 finely chopped
1 tsp Dijon mustard
2 tbsp olive oil

FOR THE TOMATOES
4 sprays of cherry tomatoes on
 the vine (4-5 on each one)
a few sprigs of basil

Some of us, me included, can be a little nervous about cooking fish. I'm torn on which method is best, but this is a really easy option. The fish is coated with a lovely crunchy crust and baked in the oven, then served with a cheesy sauce. You can't go wrong. I like to serve some greens and sautéed potatoes with the fish.

First, make the cheese sauce. Heat the butter in a saucepan and add the flour. Stir until it has combined into a paste, then cook for 3 to 4 minutes, stirring constantly, to cook out the flavour of raw flour. Add a little milk and stir – you will find it thickens up very quickly and, as you stir, will come away from the base of the pan. Add the remaining milk, very gradually to start with and stirring or whisking thoroughly after each addition, until you have a smooth, pourable sauce. Stir in the Cheddar and mustard and taste for seasoning. Add salt and pepper as necessary.

To prepare the cod, preheat the oven to 200°C (180°C fan)/gas 6 and line a roasting tin with baking parchment.

Make the crust by mixing together the breadcrumbs, capers, gherkins or jalapeños, herbs, mustard and oil, then season with pepper – it should be salty enough because of the olives and capers.

Divide the crust mixture among the four pieces of cod and press lightly onto the flesh. Arrange in the roasting tin and add the sprays of cherry tomatoes. Roast in the oven for around 15 minutes until the cod is cooked through, the crust lightly browned and the tomatoes plump and close to bursting.

Reheat the cheese sauce and give it a good whisk to make sure it is smooth, then serve with the cod, tomatoes and a few sprigs of basil, perhaps with some potatoes and cooked greens on the side.

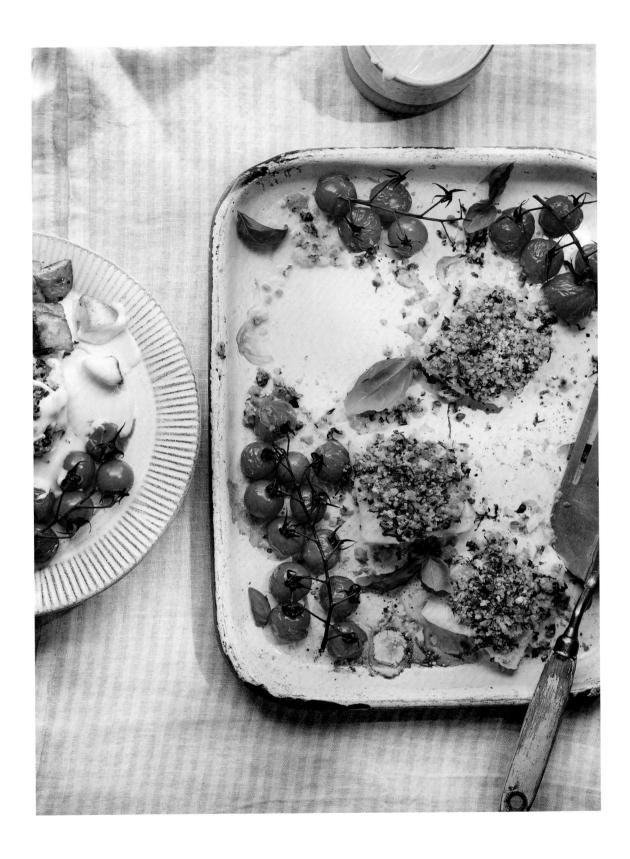

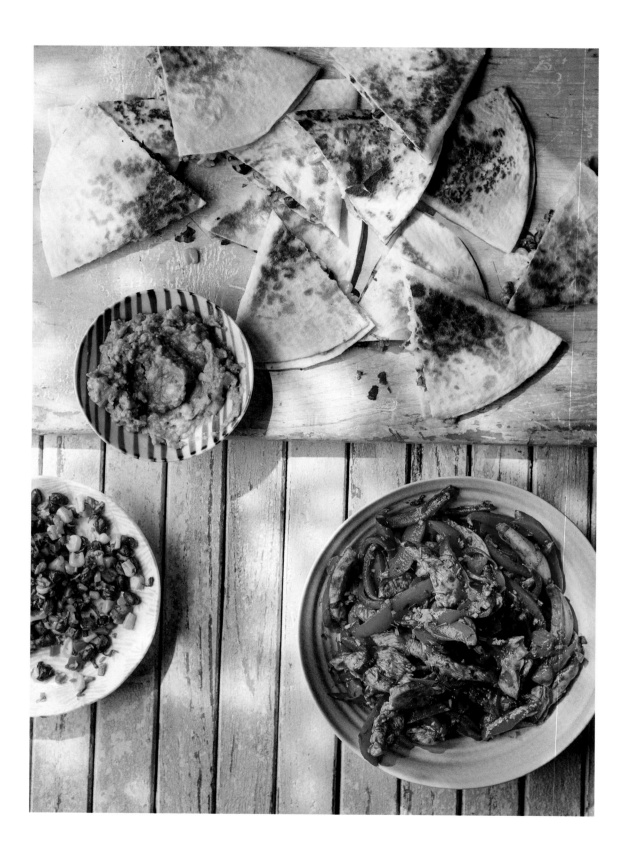

Quesadillas are a real family favourite and everyone can choose their own optional extras – avocados, jalapeños, grated cheese, pineapple (of course!) and so on. You don't need a lot of chicken – in fact, you could leave it out altogether and add more green vegetables, such as sprouting broccoli, as there is plenty of protein in the beans and cheese.

Fajita-style Chicken + Vegetables with Quesadillas

Put the chicken breasts in a bowl and season with salt and pepper. Sprinkle over the lime juice and zest and leave to stand while you prepare the vegetables.

Heat the olive oil in a large sauté pan. Add the red onion and peppers. Cook on a fairly high heat until starting to brown, but still quite firm. Add the chicken and continue to cook until the chicken is browned on all sides. Add the garlic for the last couple of minutes.

Stir in the spices, chipotle paste and tomato and season with salt and pepper. Add a splash of water and cook over a high heat until the chicken is completely cooked through. Keep warm.

To make the quesadillas, mix together the beans, sweetcorn, jalapeños, if using, and coriander. Season with salt and pepper. If using the avocado, mix with the lime juice. Spread each half of the tortillas with the avocado, then top with 2 heaped tablespoons of the bean mix. Sprinkle over the cheese and fold over. Repeat with the remaining tortillas until you have six folded.

Heat a large frying pan and cook the quesadillas on a medium heat for a few minutes on each side until they are lightly browned with the cheese melting and hot. Cut each quesadilla into four wedges and serve on the side with the chicken and vegetables, garnished with a few sprigs of coriander.

PREP 25 MINS
COOK ABOUT 35 MINS
SERVES 4

FOR THE CHICKEN + VEGETABLES
2 chicken breasts, cut into strips
zest and juice of ½ lime
1 tbsp olive oil
2 red onions, cut into wedges
2 peppers, cut into strips
3 garlic cloves, finely chopped
½ tsp ground cumin
½ tsp ground cinnamon
2 tsp chipotle paste
1 tomato, diced
a few sprigs of coriander
salt and black pepper

FOR THE QUESADILLAS
1 × 400g (14oz) tin black beans, drained
200g (7oz) frozen sweetcorn, defrosted
2 tbsp pickled jalapeños, roughly chopped (optional)
a few sprigs of chopped coriander
2 avocados, mashed (optional)
juice of ½ lime (optional)
6 large tortillas, preferably corn or corn/flour combo
225g (8oz) grated Cheddar cheese

Golden Chicken Nuggets with Sweet Potato Mash

PREP 25 MINS, PLUS MARINATING
COOK ABOUT 30 MINS
SERVES 4

FOR THE CHICKEN NUGGETS
zest and juice of 1 lime
2 garlic cloves, crushed or grated
2 tbsp thick live yoghurt
3 chicken breasts, diced or cut into strips
½–1 tsp smoked paprika
½ tsp curry powder (optional)
75g (3oz) panko or similar breadcrumbs
1 tbsp sesame seeds (optional)
oil, for brushing
salt and black pepper

FOR THE SWEET POTATO MASH
200g (7oz) floury potatoes, peeled and cut into chunks
400g (14oz) sweet potatoes, peeled and cut into chunks
25g (1oz) butter

FOR THE DIP
250g (9oz) thick live yoghurt
3 tbsp mango chutney
1 tsp hot sauce (optional)
a few sprigs of coriander, finely chopped

These are so much tastier than anything shop-bought and way healthier. The yoghurt marinade is good for gut health and it is well worth adding the sesame seeds to the breadcrumb coating, as they provide extra fibre and nutrients – my kids don't even notice them! The sweet potato mash, made with half sweet and half regular potatoes, is an ideal accompaniment and more nutritious than white potato mash.

Put the lime juice and zest, garlic and yoghurt in a bowl with ½ teaspoon salt and some black pepper. Toss the chicken breasts in the mixture and cover and leave to marinate for half an hour.

Preheat your oven to 200°C (180°C fan)/gas 6.

Remove the chicken from the marinade, wiping off any excess, then toss in the smoked paprika and curry powder, if using. Put the breadcrumbs and sesame seeds in a shallow bowl with a little more salt and pepper. Dip the chicken pieces in this mixture, making sure they are well covered, and arrange over a baking tray. Brush the nuggets with oil and bake for around 15 minutes until cooked through and a crisp rich brown.

For the sweet potato mash, put all the potatoes in a lidded steamer basket over simmering water and steam until tender, about 15 minutes. Mash with the butter and season to taste.

For the dip, put the yoghurt in a bowl and add salt and pepper. If the mango chutney is very chunky, chop it so it is more uniform, then add to the yoghurt along with the hot sauce, if using, and coriander. Mix thoroughly. Serve with the chicken and mash and maybe some corn on the cob or peas.

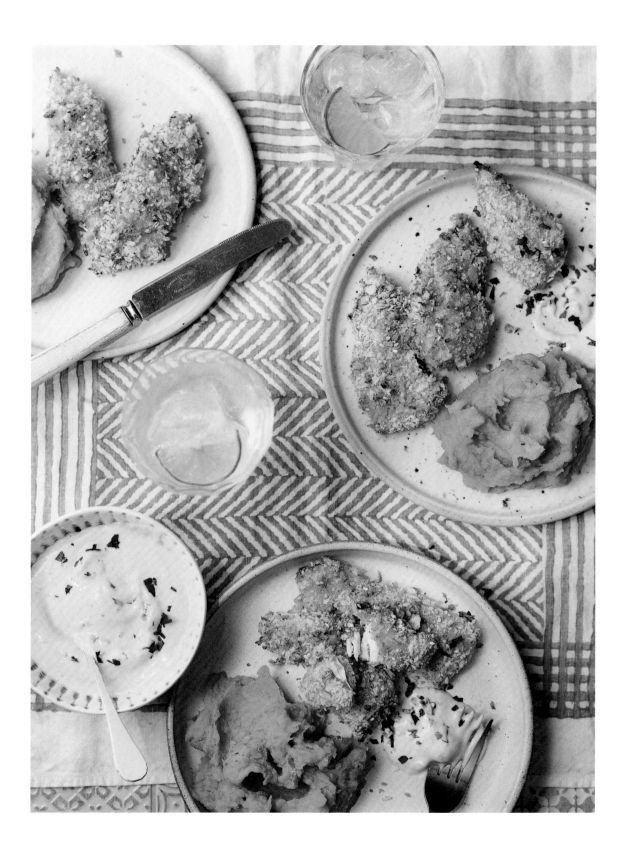

Soul-soothing Chicken Pie

PREP 30 MINS, PLUS CHILLING
COOK ABOUT 1 HOUR 10 MINS
SERVES 4

Chicken pie always tastes like home to me – it's like a comfort blanket, a toasty fire and a back rub all at once, if you get me. It's absolutely delicious on its own or with sides of minted peas and rustic mashed potato. Use chicken breast or thigh meat – whichever you prefer – and there are plenty of vegetables in there too, including carrots, which bring a lovely sweetness to the pie.

First, make the pastry. Put the flour in a bowl with a generous pinch of salt and add the butter. Rub the butter into the flour until it resembles fine breadcrumbs. Add the egg and just enough iced water to make a firm dough. Make sure it isn't flaky as this will make it harder to roll. Wrap or put in a container and chill for 30 minutes.

To make the filling, put the carrots with a knob of the butter and a pinch of salt in a saucepan and just cover with water. Bring to the boil, then cover and simmer until tender – around 7 to 8 minutes. Drain and set aside to cool.

Meanwhile, melt the oil and remaining butter in a large, lidded sauté pan. Add the chicken and cook until the surface area is cooked. Stir in the leeks and garlic, making sure they are well covered with the butter, then season with salt and pepper. Add the wine, tarragon sprigs and bay leaves. Bring to the boil, then cover and turn down the heat. Leave to braise until the chicken is cooked through and leeks are tender – around 10 minutes.

Remove the chicken, herbs and leeks from the pan and measure the remaining liquid into a jug. Discard the tarragon sprigs and bay leaves. Add enough chicken stock to bring it up to 300ml (10½fl oz), then pour into a saucepan. Whisk the cornflour with 50ml (1¾fl oz) cold water, then add to the chicken stock mixture. Slowly heat, bringing to the boil and whisking until the mixture thickens to the consistency of a béchamel sauce. Remove from the heat and stir in the crème fraîche and mustard, if using.

Mix the sauce with the chicken, leeks and carrots and leave to cool completely.

To assemble and bake, remove the pastry from the fridge half an hour before you want to use it. Preheat the oven to 200°C (180°C fan)/gas 6.

Lightly flour a work surface. Take two-thirds of the pastry dough and roll it out into a round. Use it to line the base of a pie dish, about 21cm (8½ inches) across and 5cm (2 inches) deep, and add the filling.

Roll out the remainder of the pastry. Brush the edges of the bottom layer of pastry with egg wash, then add the top layer. Trim the edges, then crimp together with finger or thumb or fork prongs. Cut two slits in the middle, then brush generously with the egg wash.

Put on a baking tray and bake for 30 to 35 minutes until the pastry is golden brown and the filling is piping hot.

FOR THE PASTRY

350g (12oz) plain flour
a generous pinch of salt
175g (6oz) butter, chilled
　and diced
1 egg, beaten
iced water

FOR THE FILLING

300g (10½oz) large carrots,
　sliced at an angle
20g (¾oz) butter
1 tbsp olive oil
600g (1lb 5oz) chicken, diced
3 leeks, cut into rounds
3 garlic cloves, finely chopped
100ml (3½fl oz) white wine
2 sprigs of tarragon
2 bay leaves
up to 300ml (10½fl oz) chicken
　stock
1½ tbsp cornflour
50g (1¾oz) crème fraîche
2 tsp Dijon or tarragon mustard
　(optional)
salt and black pepper

1 egg, beaten for an egg wash

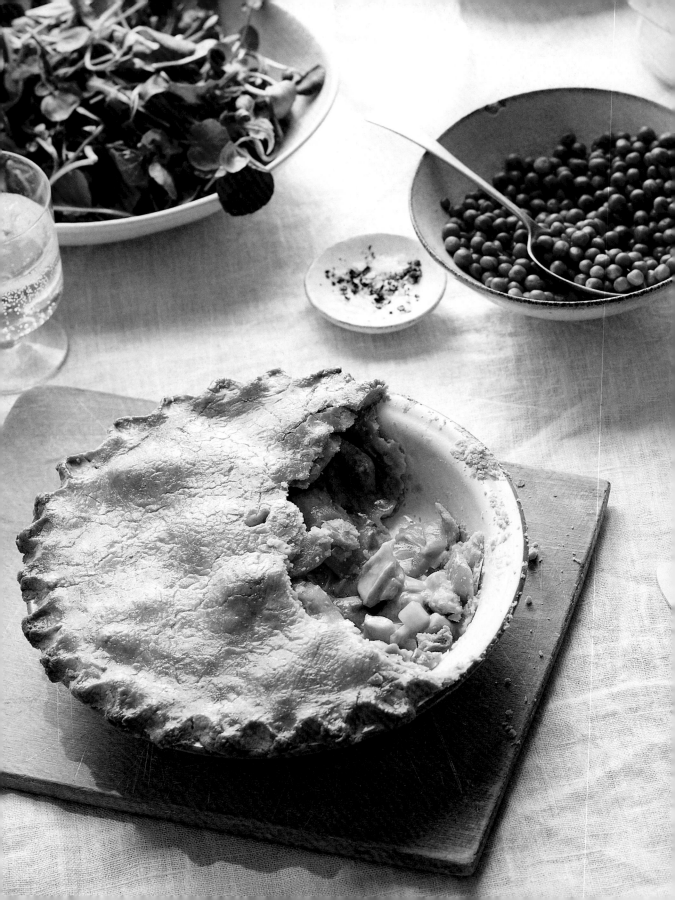

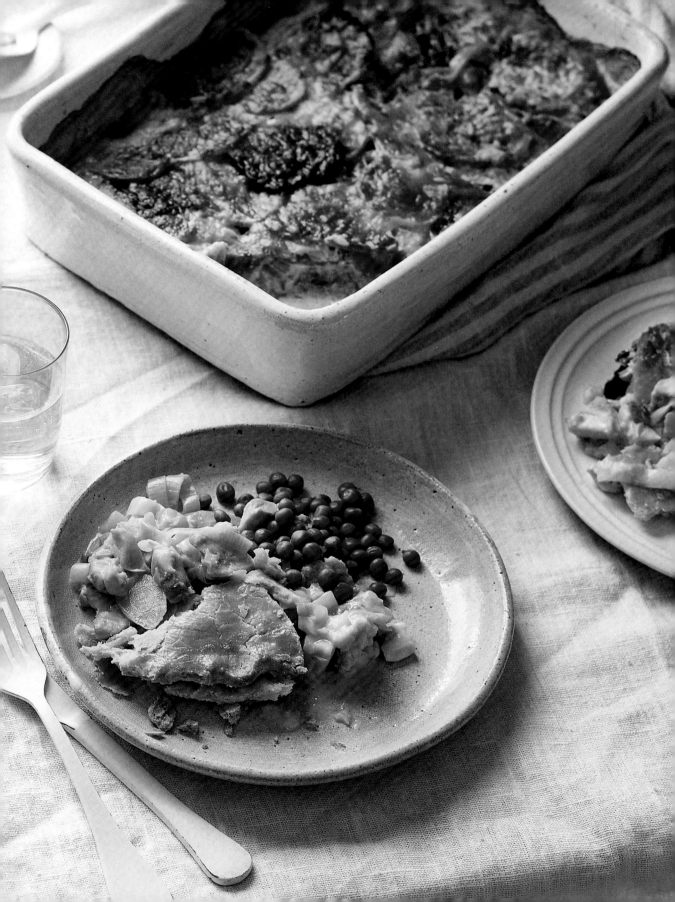

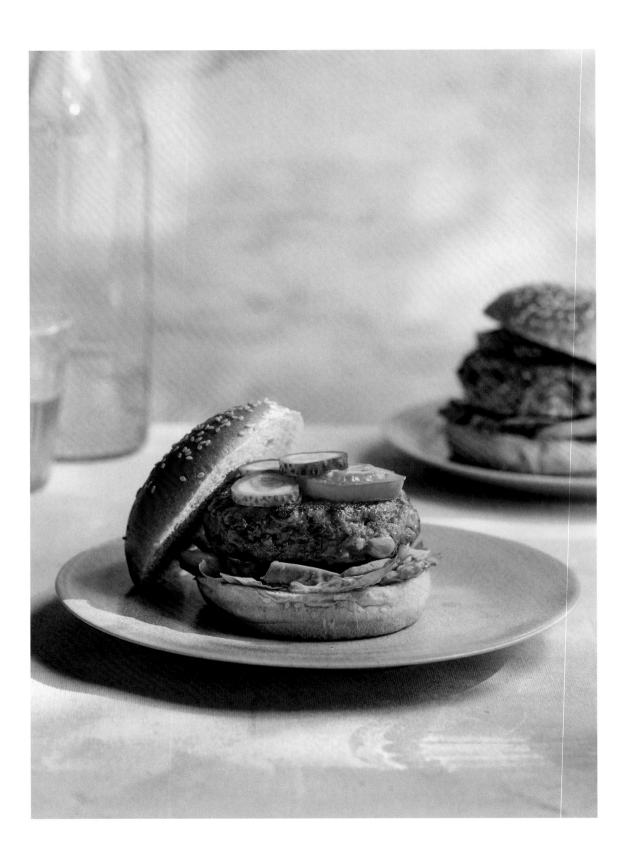

Turkey is much lower in fat than beef mince yet so tasty that I use it for burgers. I buy turkey mince and add breadcrumbs, yoghurt and some egg to keep the burgers succulent, not dry. They are quite substantial and you can make the mixture into six smaller portions if you prefer. The sweetcorn and peas add a little sweetness and texture. The family love getting involved in building their own burgers and adding different toppings, such as avocado, jalapeños, salad and cheese.

First, make the burgers. Heat half the oil in a frying pan and add the onion. Sauté on a medium-low heat until the onion is soft and translucent, then add the garlic. Stir for another minute or two, then remove from the heat and leave to cool down.

Put the turkey mince in a bowl with the onion and garlic mixture and all the remaining burger ingredients. Season well and mix thoroughly. The easiest way to do this is with your hands. The mixture will feel very soft to start with – keep turning it over in your hands and lightly kneading it until it starts to feel firmer.

Divide the mixture into four and shape into large patties. Chill in the fridge for an hour if possible – this will make them easier to handle when you cook them.

When you're ready to cook the burgers, remove them from the fridge. Heat the remaining oil in a large frying pan and add the burgers, well-spaced out. Fry for several minutes on each side – you will know when they are ready to flip as they will look cooked up the sides and will come away cleanly from the pan. Make sure they are completely cooked through (if you have a probe thermometer, they should read 72°C/162°F, or if you insert the tip of a knife, it should be almost too hot to press between your fingers for longer than a second).

If adding the cheese, arrange over the burgers and cover with a lid to help it melt.

To assemble, toss the avocado with the lime juice. Place a burger on the bottom half of a bun, then top with the avocado, jalapeños, salad leaves and tomato. Serve with any other condiments you like.

Tess's Tremendous Turkey Burgers

PREP 20 MINS, PLUS CHILLING
COOK ABOUT 20 MINS
SERVES 4

FOR THE BURGERS
2 tbsp olive oil
1 small onion, very
    finely chopped
4 garlic cloves, crushed
500g (1lb 2oz) turkey mince
50g (1¾oz) frozen sweetcorn,
    defrosted
50g (1¾oz) frozen peas,
    defrosted
a few sprigs of coriander, very
    finely chopped
50g (1¾oz) breadcrumbs
    (preferably wholemeal)
25g (1oz) thick live yoghurt
1 egg
salt and black pepper

TO ASSEMBLE
50g (1¾oz) Cheddar cheese or
    similar, grated (optional)
1 large avocado, peeled
    and sliced
juice of 1 lime
4 burger buns or large
    lettuce leaves
2 tbsp pickled jalapeños
a few salad leaves
1 large tomato, thinly sliced

Rainbow Veggie Traybake

Packed with colourful vegetables, this traybake is a feast for the eye as well as being tasty and good for the gut. I like to add some beans for protein and black beans are particularly high in fibre and nutrients.

PREP 20 MINS
COOK 40 MINS
SERVES 4

FOR THE TRAYBAKE

2 red onions, cut into wedges

3 peppers (any colour), cut into thick slices

500g (1lb 2oz) squash, cut into wedges (no need to peel)

2 tbsp olive oil

1 large head of broccoli, cut into florets

1 × 400g (14oz) tin of black beans, drained (optional)

200g (7oz) frozen sweetcorn, defrosted

4 spring onions, sliced into rounds

300g (10½oz) cherry tomatoes

a few sprigs of coriander

salt and black pepper

FOR THE SAUCE

1 tbsp red wine vinegar

1 tbsp soy sauce

juice of 1 lime

1 tsp honey

2 red chillies, finely chopped

2 garlic cloves, crushed

FOR THE YOGHURT DRESSING

250g (9oz) thick live yoghurt

juice of ½ lime

1 tsp honey

1 tsp chipotle paste

a pinch of ground cinnamon

a few sprigs of coriander, finely chopped

FOR THE SMASHED AVOCADO

juice of 1 lime

a generous pinch of salt

2 avocados, roughly mashed/smashed

Preheat the oven to 200°C (180°C fan)/gas 6.

Put the onion, peppers and squash in a large roasting tin. Drizzle over a tablespoon of the oil, then season with salt and pepper. Roast in the oven for 15 minutes. Toss the broccoli in the remaining oil and add to the roasting tin. Cover with foil and return to the oven to cook for a further 10 minutes.

Add the black beans and sweetcorn to the roasting tin, giving it all a good shake to make sure they fall to the bottom.

Whisk all the sauce ingredients together and drizzle this over the roasting tin, making sure you give it another good shake as you do so. Season with salt and pepper again, then sprinkle over the spring onion and cherry tomatoes.

Return to the oven and cook for around another 15 minutes until all the vegetables are tender and the tomatoes are close to bursting. Remove from the oven and garnish with coriander leaves.

For the yoghurt dressing, mix the yoghurt, lime juice, honey, chipotle and cinnamon together and stir in plenty of chopped coriander. Season with salt and pepper.

For the smashed avocado, put the lime juice in a bowl with a generous pinch of salt and add the avocado. Mix thoroughly.

Serve the traybake with the yoghurt dressing and smashed avocado on the side.

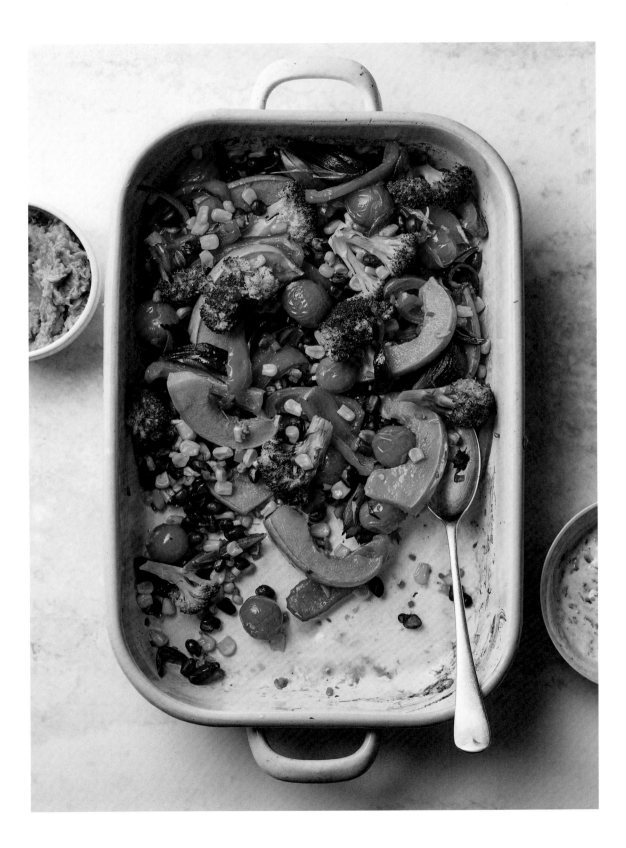

Fabulous Fried Rice

PREP 15 MINS
COOK ABOUT 10 MINS
SERVES 4

1 tbsp vegetable oil
1 large carrot, cut into sticks
100g (3½oz) broccoli, chopped
300g (10½oz) mixed
   mushrooms (shiitake, button
   or chestnut), roughly chopped
1 red onion, finely chopped
100g (3½oz) sliced baby corn
100g (3½oz) frozen sweetcorn,
   defrosted
1 courgette, diced
200g (7oz) frozen peas,
   defrosted
500g (1lb 2oz) cooked rice
   (175–200g/6–7oz uncooked)

FOR THE SAUCE
1 tsp sesame oil
3 tbsp soy sauce
1 tbsp mirin
1 tsp honey or kecap manis
   (sweetened soy sauce)
1 red chilli, finely chopped
10g (¼oz) root ginger, grated
2 garlic cloves, grated
½ tsp Chinese 5 spice

TO SERVE
1 tsp sesame seeds
a small bunch of coriander,
   chopped
chilli oil or chilli flakes

An easy supper dish, this is loaded with vegetables and mushrooms, which I've discovered are really beneficial for the gut. You can add any leftover cooked veg you have in the fridge, such as green beans, broccoli or cabbage and even a little leftover meat. Just a tiny amount gives a flavour boost and can be added with the mushrooms. The sauce, sweetened with honey, is delicious and the fresh root ginger and garlic ups the nutritional content.

First, make the sauce. Mix all the ingredients together with 50ml (1¾fl oz) water.

Heat the oil in your wok or a large sauté pan. Add the carrot and broccoli and cook on a high heat until starting to soften and brown. Add the mushrooms, red onion, baby corn, sweetcorn, courgette and peas. Continue to stir-fry on a high heat until the vegetables are just cooked through.

Pour over the sauce. Allow to bubble up, then stir quickly to coat all the vegetables. Finally, stir in the rice. Keep stir-frying until the rice is piping hot.

Serve sprinkled with the seeds and coriander. Increase the heat by adding chilli oil or chilli flakes at the table.

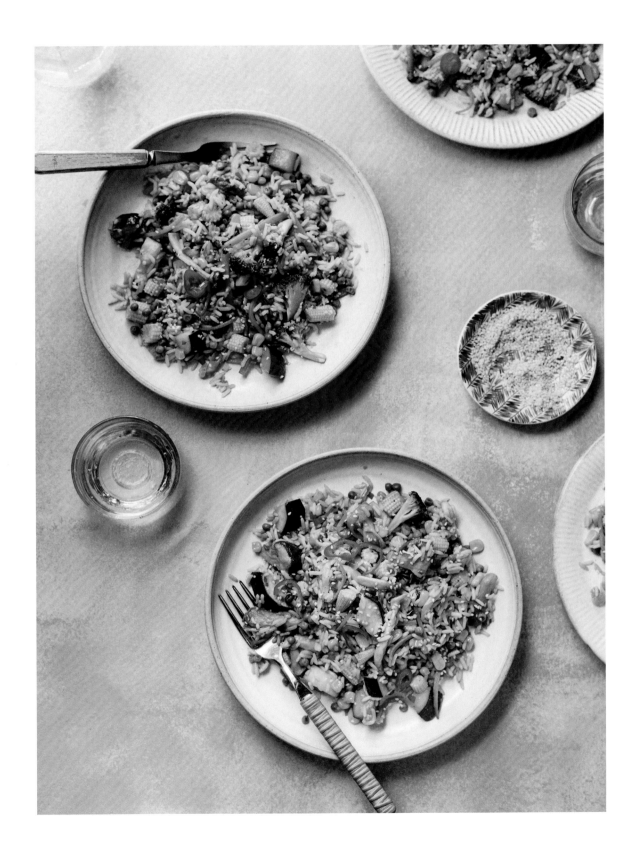

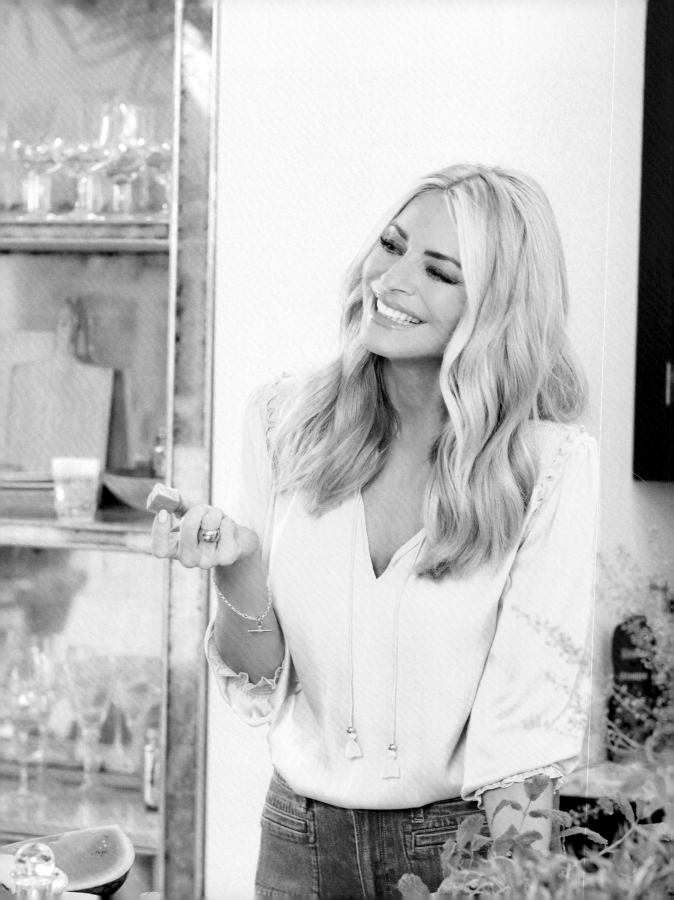

DESSERTS

A little of what you fancy does you good

Totally Tropical Fruit Salad

PREP 15 MINS, PLUS CHILLING
COOK LESS THAN 10 MINS
SERVES 4

FOR THE SYRUP
50g (1¾oz) honey
zest and juice of 1 lime
5g (⅛oz) root ginger, sliced
½ tsp black peppercorns
½ tsp allspice berries
3cm (1¼ inch) piece of
  cinnamon stick (optional)

FOR THE FRUIT SALAD
1 large mango, peeled
  and diced
250g (9oz) pineapple, peeled
  and diced
½ green melon, peeled,
  deseeded and diced
pulp and seeds from
  1 passion fruit
1–2 bananas, peeled and diced
  (optional)
1 papaya, peeled, deseeded
  and diced, or another mango
  or one of the other fruits

TO GARNISH
a few mint leaves
a very fine grating of nutmeg

Tropical fruits like mango and pineapple are beautifully sweet already, so I just use a little honey in the syrup for this salad and some tasty spices to make the flavours really sing. If serving this for grown-ups, you could add a spoonful of rum as well.

First, make the syrup – this can and should be made ahead so the flavours have time to infuse and for the syrup to chill. Put the honey, lime zest, ginger, peppercorns, allspice and cinnamon, if using, into a small saucepan with 100ml (3½fl oz) water. Heat over a low heat, stirring until the honey has dissolved, then bring to the boil and remove from the heat. Leave to cool, then strain and add the lime juice. Chill for a couple of hours or overnight.

Put all the fruit salad ingredients in a bowl and drizzle over a couple of tablespoons of the syrup. Keep in the fridge until ready to serve. Garnish with a few mint leaves and a fine grating of nutmeg.

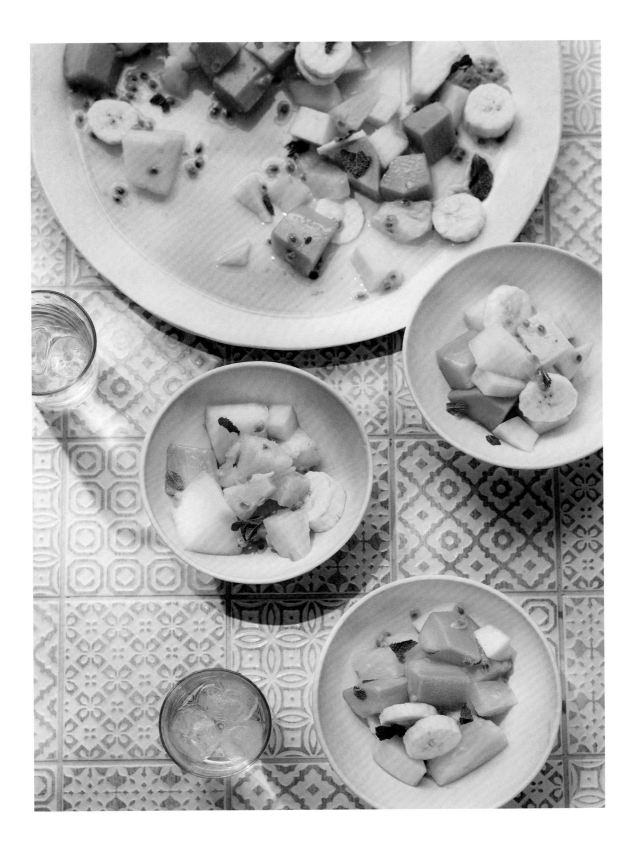

My Sister's Instant Ice Cream Sundaes

PREP 10 MINS, PLUS FREEZING
COOK ABOUT 5 MINS
SERVES 4

FOR THE ICE CREAM
3 large ripe bananas
juice of ½ lime
2 tbsp honey or maple syrup
50g (1¾oz) thick live yoghurt

FOR THE NUTS
100g (3½oz) nuts (any, mixed
   is good)
1 tbsp maple syrup or honey
a pinch of salt
a pinch of ground cinnamon

TO ASSEMBLE
400g (14oz) mixture of berries,
   any large strawberries halved
300ml (10½fl oz) whipping or
   double cream (or squeezy
   aerosol cream if you prefer)

OPTIONAL EXTRAS
any leftover cake that might be
   lying around would be good
   diced and put in as a layer for
   an extra treat

My sister Karen lives in New Zealand and shared this recipe with me and I've loved it ever since. There's no such thing as convenience foods there, so you've no choice but to make pretty much everything from scratch! The ice cream for these is simple to make but needs a little advance prep – you'll have to freeze the bananas a few hours before, or preferably overnight. Once that's done, the rest is a breeze.

A few hours (or the day before) you want to make this ice cream, cut the bananas into chunks and toss in the lime juice. Arrange on a baking tray or put in a freezer bag and freeze until solid.

Put the frozen bananas in a food processor with the lime juice, honey or maple syrup and yoghurt. Blitz until the bananas have broken down into a thick, smooth ice cream. Put into Tupperware and return to the freezer until you're ready to use it.

Put the nuts in a dry frying pan and toast on a medium heat until they start to lightly colour and smell aromatic. Drizzle over the maple syrup or honey along with a pinch of salt and the cinnamon. Continue to fry, stirring constantly, until the nuts are well coated and glossy. Keep stirring until the honey or maple syrup looks dry – it will eventually crystallize around the nuts. Remove from the heat and leave to cool, then roughly crush.

To make the sundaes, put a couple of tablespoons of berries in the base of each sundae glass or bowl. Top with a scoop of the ice cream and follow with the remaining fruit. Add a generous dollop of cream, then sprinkle over the nuts. Serve immediately.

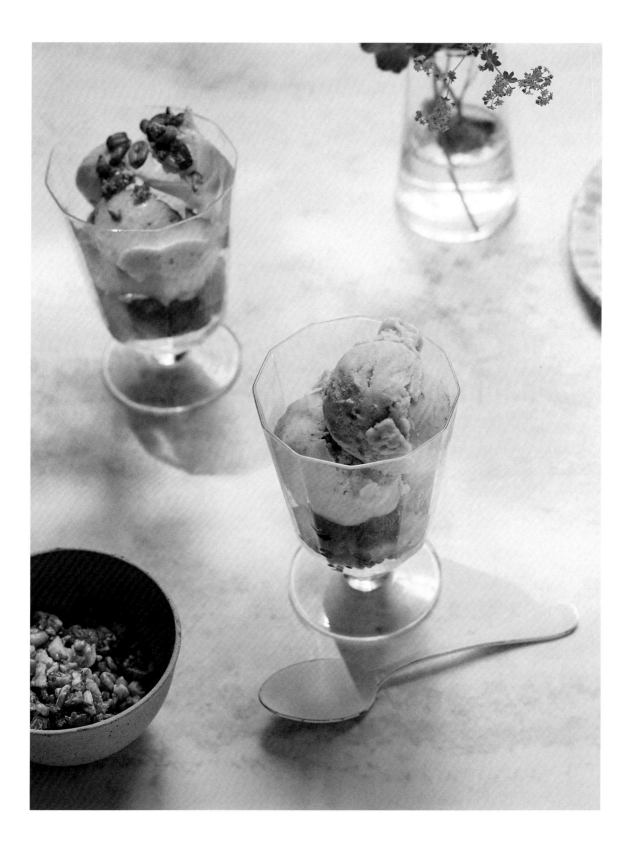

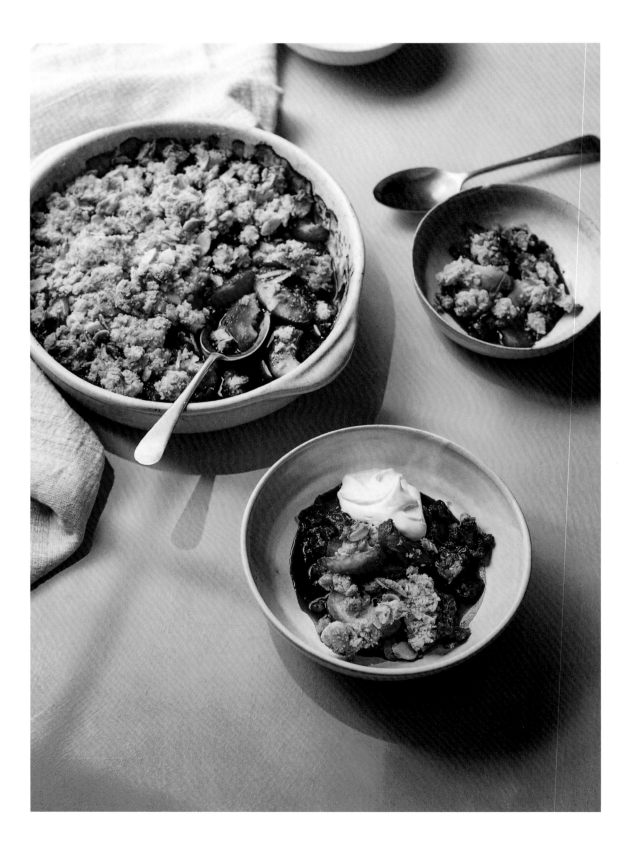

Scrumptious Peach + Almond Crumble

This crumble is healthier than your average one. I love the combo of peaches and blueberries in this crumble, but you could also use nectarines or plums if you prefer. Just make sure they are quite ripe but not too soft. The topping contains oats and almonds to boost fibre and protein content and the gentle spicing helps to add a bit of sweetness as I've reduced the usual amount of sugar.

PREP 15 MINS
COOK ABOUT 25 MINS
SERVES 4

4 peaches or nectarines
1 tbsp light soft brown sugar or maple syrup
150g (5½oz) blueberries (optional)

FOR THE TOPPING
50g (1¾oz) plain flour (spelt, rye and wholemeal are all good)
50g (1¾oz) ground almonds
50g (1¾oz) porridge oats
½ tsp mixed spice or ground cinnamon or ground cardamom
a pinch of salt
75g (3oz) butter, chilled and diced
50g (1¾oz) flaked almonds
50ml (1¾fl oz) maple syrup
2 tsp demerara sugar (optional)

Preheat the oven to 200°C (180°C fan)/gas 6 and butter an ovenproof dish.

Cut the peaches or nectarines into wedges, discarding the stones as you go. Toss with the sugar or maple syrup and arrange with the blueberries, if using, over the base of the dish.

Put the flour and ground almonds in a bowl with the porridge oats and any spices you might want to use, along with a pinch of salt. Add the butter and rub in, then stir in the flaked almonds and maple syrup. You will find that it clumps together quite a bit, but this is fine. Sprinkle over the peaches as evenly as you can, then sprinkle over the demerara sugar for extra crunch.

Bake in the oven for around 25 minutes until the peaches are soft and the topping crisp and golden brown.

Hit-me-up Power Balls

PREP 10 MINS, PLUS CHILLING
MAKES 12 BALLS

125g (4½oz) crunchy nut butter
  (any sort)
85g (3oz) honey
a few drops of vanilla extract
50g (1¾oz) porridge oats
25g (1oz) desiccated coconut
25g (1oz) sesame seeds
15g (½oz) chia seeds
10g (¼oz) milled flax seeds
a pinch of salt

FOR THE COATING

15g (½oz) of sesame seeds,
  desiccated coconut, cocoa or
  finely chopped nuts

There are lots of great nutrients and plenty of fibre in these little energy boosters, so they are super-good for you. Chia seeds are particularly beneficial for gut health and contain omega-3 fats as well as vitamins and minerals. These are perfect as an after-school snack, and I eat a couple on the way to the gym if I've not had time for breakfast.

Put the nut butter in a bowl with the honey and vanilla extract and stir to combine. Add all the dry ingredients and mix to a stiff, slightly tacky paste.

Divide into 12 pieces and shape into balls, then roll in your choice of coating. Chill for about 30 minutes or until firm. Store in the fridge in an airtight container.

VARIATIONS: To give a good chocolate hit, add 25g (1oz) cocoa to the mix or add a tablespoon of cacao nibs.

Add spices to give extra micronutrients – pinches of ground cinnamon, cardamom, turmeric (if using, add a pinch of black pepper too), ginger, allspice and/or cayenne would all work.

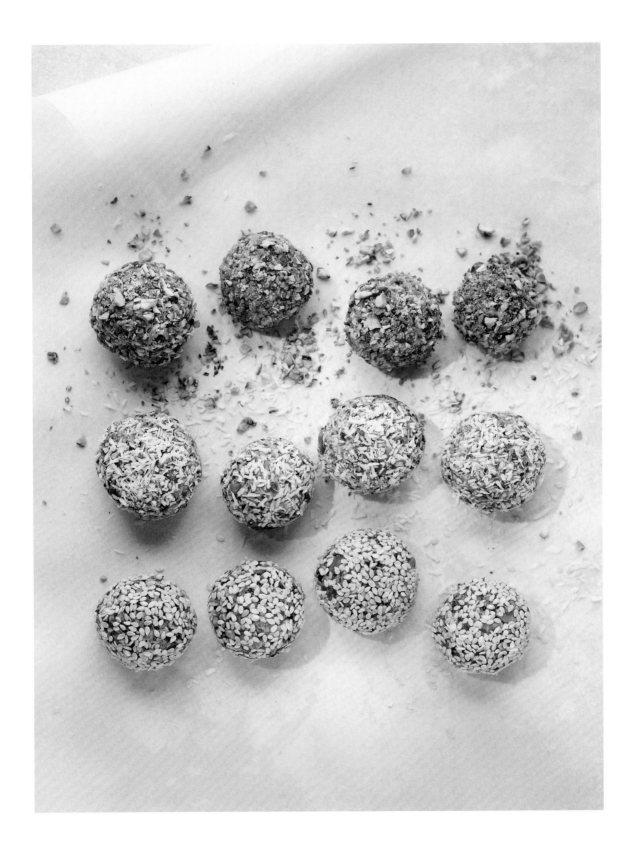

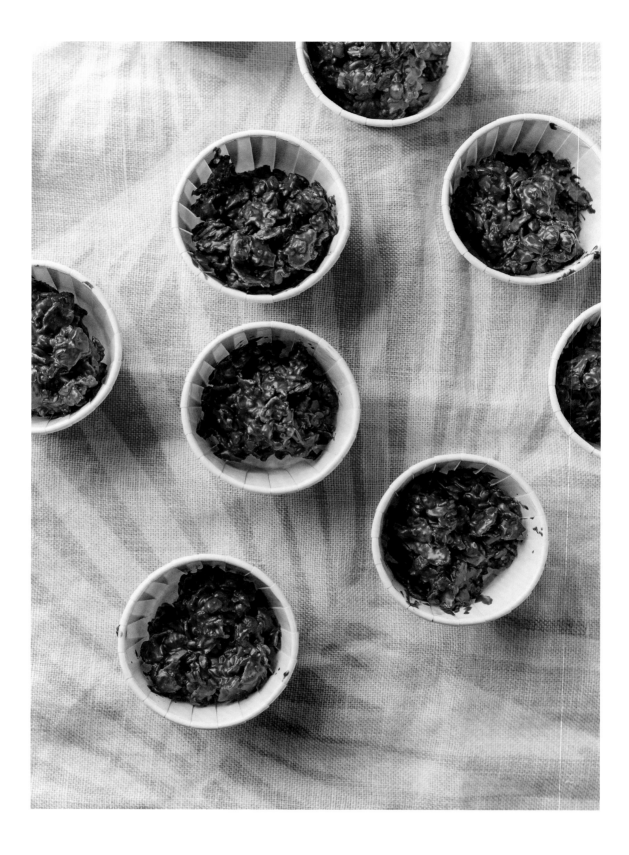

Chocolate Cornflake Cakes

The traditional version of these I used to have as a child was just made with cornflakes, but these days I like to add some oats, nuts and seeds for a healthier, crunchier treat. Initially, I thought my girls would baulk at the thought of 'messing with perfection' but now they can't get enough of them!

PREP 10 MINUTES, PLUS CHILLING
MAKES 12 CUPCAKES

200g (7oz) dark chocolate
50ml (1¾fl oz) maple syrup
50g (1¾oz) butter or coconut oil
50g (1¾oz) cornflakes
25g (1oz) porridge oats
25g (1oz) mixed nuts, chopped
  or flaked
10g (¼oz) mixed seeds
½ tsp ground ginger (optional)
¼ tsp ground cinnamon
  (optional)
¼ tsp cayenne powder
  (optional)

Put the chocolate, maple syrup and butter or coconut oil in a heatproof bowl. Set it over simmering water and stir gently until it has completely melted.

Put the cornflakes in a bowl and scrunch them lightly with your hands to break them up a bit. Stir in the oats, nuts, seeds and spices, if using. Pour over the melted chocolate mixture and thoroughly combine.

Line a 12-hole cake tin with paper cases. Divide the mixture among the cases – there should be enough for 1 heaped tablespoon per case. Chill in the fridge for about an hour until the chocolate has reset and store in an airtight container.

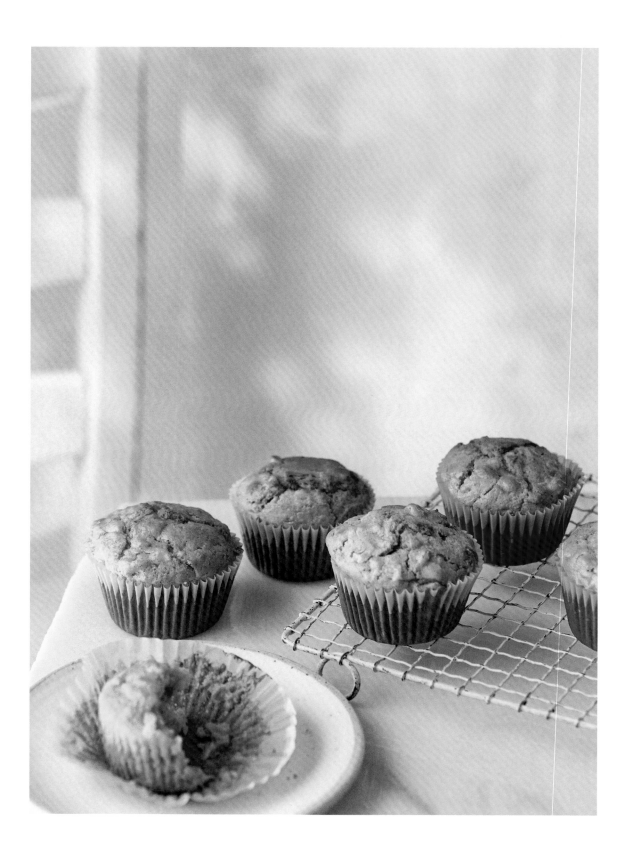

Apple +
Pecan Muffins

PREP 15 MINS
COOK 20–25 MINS
MAKES 12 MUFFINS

These are lovely at teatime or breakfast. Using some rye flour gives them a nice nutty flavour and I sweeten them with half sugar and half maple syrup, which work really well with the apples and pecans. If you prefer, make smaller muffins in fairy cake tins, in which case you'll get about twenty-four.

DRY INGREDIENTS
200g (7oz) plain flour
100g (3½oz) rye flour
2 tbsp baking powder
½ tsp bicarbonate of soda
2 tsp mixed spice
50g (1¾oz) caster sugar
50g (1¾oz) pecans, chopped
2 small eating apples, peeled
  and finely diced
1 medium carrot, grated
a pinch of salt

Preheat the oven to 200°C (180°C fan)/gas 6 and line a 12-hole muffin tray with paper cases.

Put all the dry ingredients in a bowl with a pinch of salt and mix together thoroughly.

Mix all the wet ingredients in a jug and whisk to combine. Pour the wet ingredients into the dry ingredients, keeping the mixing to the absolute minimum – the odd light streak of flour doesn't matter.

Divide the mixture among the muffin cases – you should find it is roughly 2 heaped tablespoons per muffin.

Bake in the oven for around 20 to 25 minutes until the muffins are well risen, golden brown and springy to touch. Remove from the oven and leave to cool on a wire rack.

Store in an airtight container.

WET INGREDIENTS
150g (5½oz) thick live yoghurt
100ml (3½fl oz) whole milk
50ml (1¾fl oz) light olive oil or
  melted butter
50ml (1¾fl oz) maple syrup
2 eggs

Heavenly Clementine, Almond + Blueberry Loaf Cake

PREP 15 MINS
COOK 40–45 MINS
MAKES 8–10 SLICES

125g (4½oz) thick live yoghurt
75ml (2½fl oz) olive oil
150g (5½oz) golden
  caster sugar
1 tbsp honey
3 medium eggs
zest of 2 clementines
  or mandarins
125g (4½oz) ground almonds
100g (3½oz) plain flour
2 tsp baking powder
a pinch of salt
100g (3½oz) blueberries

We all like a treat from time to time – and quite frankly, a day doesn't go by when I don't indulge in something sweet. If you bake your own cakes, you can be sure they are reasonably healthy. This one is made with oil and yoghurt instead of butter and I've really cut down on the sugar without compromising on taste. Simple and quick with a fragrant flavour of almonds and citrus, this makes a lovely teatime treat.

Preheat the oven to 180°C (160°C fan)/gas 4 and line a 900g (2lb) loaf tin with baking parchment.

Measure the yoghurt, oil, sugar, honey, eggs and clementine or mandarin zest into a large mixing bowl and stir well.

Mix the ground almonds, flour and baking powder in a separate bowl together with a pinch of salt. Add the dry ingredients to the wet, then fold them together gently to make a smooth batter.

Pour half the batter into the prepared loaf tin, then dot with half the blueberries. Repeat to use up the rest of the batter and berries.

Bake the cake for 40 to 45 minutes until well risen and golden brown. Leave for 5 minutes, then remove it from the tin and place on a wire rack. Serve warm or cold on its own or with yoghurt or crème fraîche.

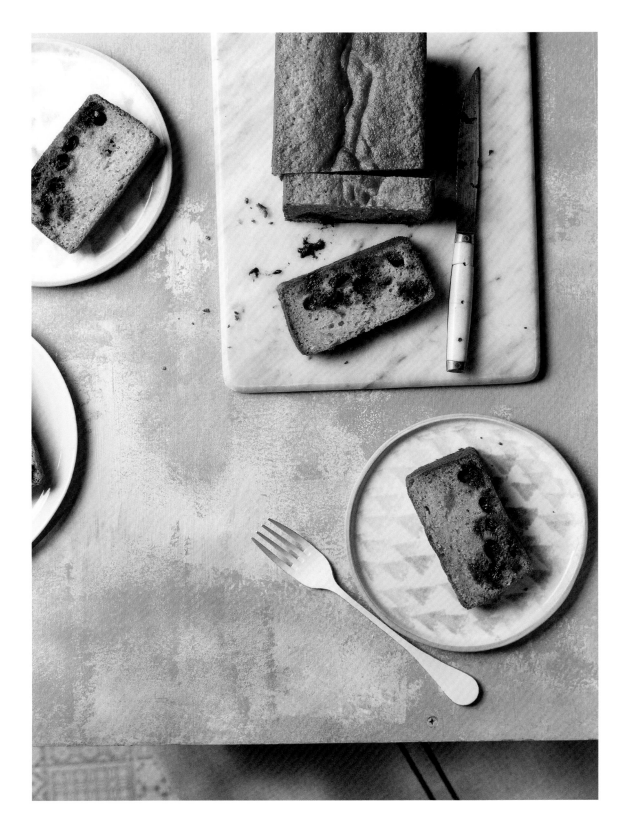

Hummingbird Cake

PREP 25 MINS, PLUS CHILLING
COOK 25–30 MINS
MAKES 1 CAKE

250g (9oz) self-raising flour
½ tsp baking powder
a generous pinch of salt
3 medium eggs
75g (3oz) light soft brown sugar
75ml (3fl oz) maple syrup
1 tsp vanilla extract
zest of 1 lime
175ml (6fl oz) sunflower oil
3 bananas, mashed
150g (5½oz) pineapple, finely
chopped (tinned is fine)
50g (1¾oz) walnuts or pecans,
finely chopped

FOR THE CREAM CHEESE ICING
50g (1¾oz) butter
75ml (3fl oz) maple syrup
zest of ½ lime
a few drops of vanilla extract
200g (7oz) cream cheese

TO GARNISH (OPTIONAL)
50g (1¾oz) walnuts or pecans,
very finely chopped

This is a beautiful cake with a nice tropical lilt from the pineapple and banana. As with all my cake recipes, I've cut down on the sugar content, but you really don't notice – it still tastes great. Some maple syrup and a little lime zest lift the cream cheese icing to something special.

Preheat the oven to 180°C (160°C fan)/gas 4. Line two 20cm (8 inch) round tins with baking parchment.

Put the flour and baking powder in a bowl with a generous pinch of salt and mix thoroughly.

Put the eggs, sugar, maple syrup, vanilla extract and lime zest into a bowl or stand mixer and whisk until very foamy – almost the consistency of mousse. Beat in the sunflower oil, followed by the flour mixture, and finally fold in the banana, pineapple and nuts.

Divide the mixture evenly between the two tins and bake for 25 to 30 minutes until well risen, springy to touch and slightly shrunken away from the tin. Remove the cakes from their tins and transfer to a wire rack to cool.

To make the icing, put the butter in a bowl or stand mixer and beat until very soft and fluffy. Add the maple syrup, lime zest and vanilla extract and beat until well combined. Add the cream cheese and mix until completely smooth with a whipped consistency. Transfer to the fridge to chill for about 20 to 30 minutes to create a firmer, spreadable consistency.

To assemble, spread some of the icing over one of the cakes and top with the other cake. Put most of the icing on top and spread it evenly. Use the rest to scrape around the sides to give an almost naked effect. Sprinkle the top with finely chopped nuts.

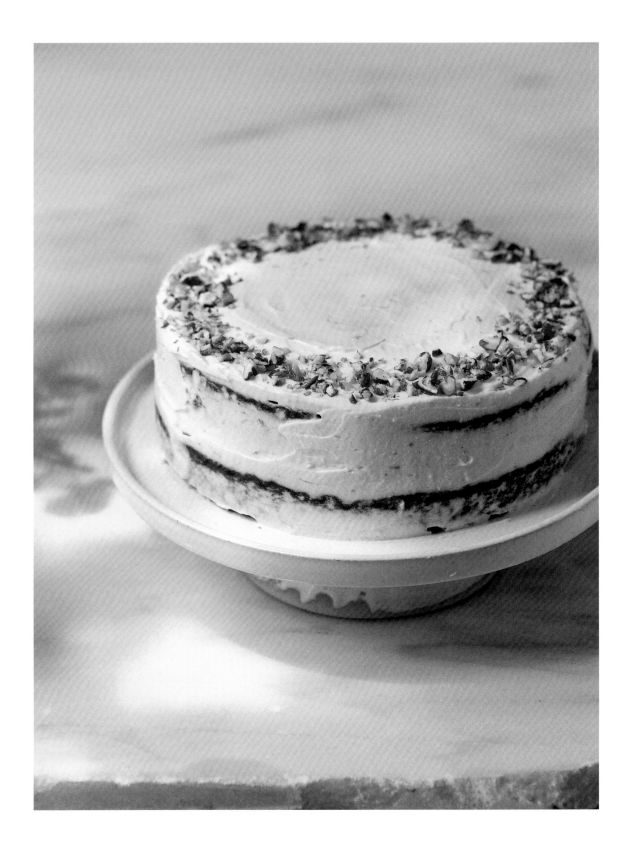

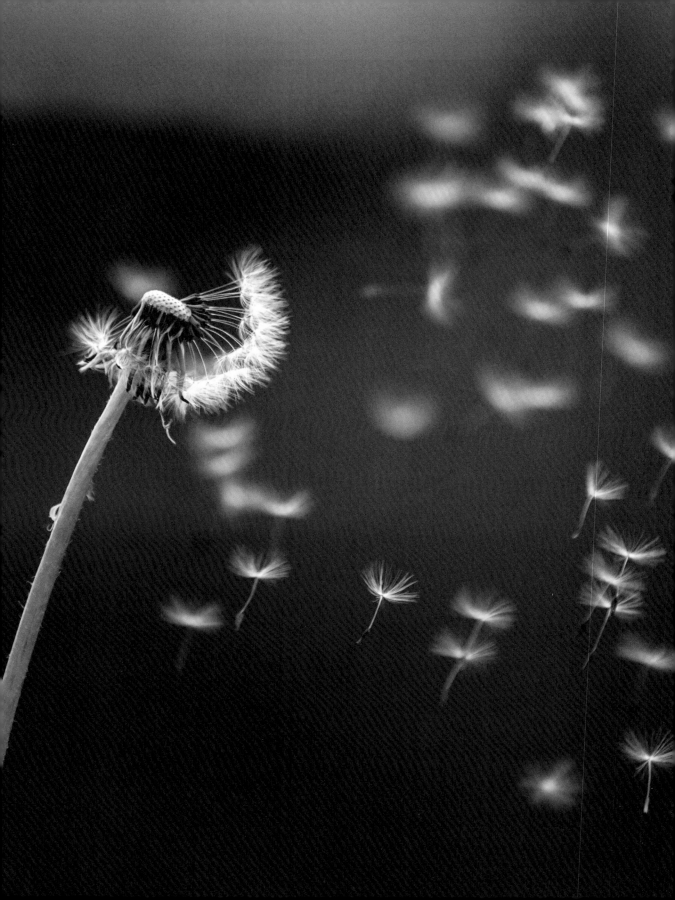

BREATHE

The way you breathe is
essential to your mental and
physical wellbeing

breathe yourself better

I have to confess that I never gave breathing much thought before. Like most of us, I've taken it for granted. But then I began to realize just how much difference focusing on my breath can make. Many people – myself included – are guilty of breathing too shallowly and therefore inefficiently.

I don't know about you, but when I discover an untapped potential source of self-improvement that lies within me and all I need to do to access its superpower is to simply, well, DO IT, it sure feels like a win. This isn't going to cost you a penny, folks. It's absolutely free. The air is there and all you have to do is B R E A T H E. To put it simply, the benefits of breathing more effectively could well change your life for the better.

Keen to know more about practical techniques to improve my breathing, I contacted breath expert and breathwork coach Rebecca Dennis. A passionate advocate of breathing properly, Rebecca has written many articles and books on the subject. She teaches practical 'conscious' breathwork techniques to improve your breathing and has been an inspiration to me on my own breath journey. And before you think, no, I can't do that – don't worry, the technique and exercises are often as simple as counting to six. You don't need any special equipment – just your breath.

the air is there and all you have to do is B R E A T H E

Rebecca fervently believes that conscious breathwork is the ultimate key to our wellbeing, health and inner calm. She's worked with thousands of people, each with their own unique needs, including autoimmune disease, chronic obstructive pulmonary disease (COPD), depression, cancer and addiction, and her clients include all sorts of people, from teachers and NHS workers to opera singers and elite athletes.

THE GOOD NEWS
IS THAT THE SIMPLE
ACT OF FOCUSING
ON THE BREATH
CAN ACTUALLY HELP
CALM AND FOCUS
THE MIND IN AN
INSTANT.

I was blown away by Rebecca's insights. Working with her, I have found new ways to relax, to feel more at home in my body and avoid getting so stressed by everyday frustrations. I've learnt a lot but I'm no expert, so she has very generously shared her knowledge and research with me to explain more about the respiratory system (in terms even I understand!) and contributed some of her exercises to help you unlock the power of breath.

As Rebecca says, 'Breathing is for everyone. It's something we all do all day, every day. You breathe in to take the oxygen needed by every cell in the body. Our breath is the instrument by which our entire respiratory system works, effectively or otherwise. It's like the starter motor for the engine that runs our entire body, and we really need it to work efficiently in order to function at our maximum capacity.'

Let's be real – it's never felt like a more appropriate time to harness the most powerful calming tool we possess, our breathing. When done right, it can greatly enhance both our physical and mental states, increasing our feeling of wellbeing and, yes, calm. The good news is that the simple act of focusing on the breath – that wondrous process of inhalation and exhalation we perform subconsciously about 23,000 times a day on average – can actually help calm and focus the mind in an instant.

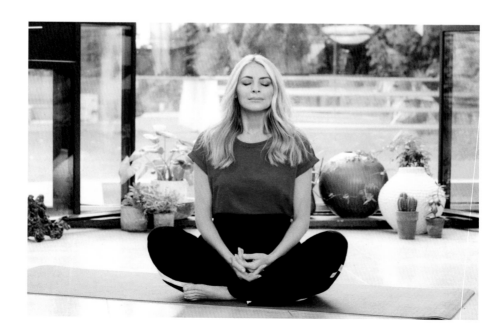

how we breathe

According to Rebecca, most adults use as little as one-third of their respiratory system. This stat alone blows my mind! Just imagine what might happen if we start using the other two-thirds! Would we become some sort of superpowered, supercharged, super-athletic version of ourselves? Because – let's be honest – that's the dream, right?!

THE BASICS OF BREATHING

'Your breath is there with you when you enter this world and breathing out will be the very last thing you do,' says Rebecca. 'You've been breathing all your life and you take it for granted because you don't have to think about it. In the same way that you blink, your heart beats and your digestive system functions, your breath is automatic.

most adults use as little as one-third of their respiratory system

'As we breathe in through the nose or mouth, air passes down through a tube in our neck called the trachea or windpipe and into the lungs. The lungs sit within the chest cavity and are protected by our ribs. At the base of the chest cavity is the diaphragm, a sheet of strong tonic muscle. When we breathe in, the diaphragm flattens, and muscles between the ribs lift the ribs up and out, allowing the lungs to expand and take air in. When we breathe out, the ribs relax and the diaphragm rises again, helping to push air out of the lungs. So good breathing involves not only the lungs but the muscles of the head, neck, chest and abdomen. Any tension in the muscles interferes with our breathing.'

TRANSFORM YOUR LIFE
THROUGH YOUR BREATH

'Breathing is a rhythmic activity,' Rebecca explains. 'Normally, the average person takes 12 to 17 breaths a minute while at rest. The rate is higher in infants and when you are in a state of excitement. It is lower when you're asleep and in those who are depressed. The depth of our breathing is another factor that varies with emotional states. Breathing becomes shallow when we are frightened or anxious. It deepens with relaxation, pleasure and sleep.

breath can be used to help with any task at hand, whether it's physical performance or mental focus

'So, when you change the way you breathe, you alter something fundamental in your whole physiology. You can change your state from feeling anxious to calm, from scattered to focused, and even from tired to more energized. Breathwork provides you with a life-long set of tools to use every day to help you navigate your way through life, and even transform it if you want to. It has been labelled by some as the 'new yoga', but it is not a replacement for anything! Better breathing can help us face, recover and heal from trauma, pain, low self-esteem and chronic anxiety.'

Rebecca has shown me that, unlike other natural functions, breath can be used to help with any task at hand, whether it's physical performance – such as diving, running or cycling – or mental focus. 'You can use your breath to physically heal yourself or to deepen your awareness,' she says. 'When you first begin to develop an awareness of your breath, it takes conscious effort and practice, but in time you'll find it easier, and it will always be there for you when you need it. The way you breathe is indicative of how you feel about life; it's no exaggeration to say it's essential to your mental and physical wellbeing.'

breathing in the body

THE DIAPHRAGM

When I started thinking more about my breath, I realized instinctively that I was not breathing deeply enough. I was rarely inhaling from my stomach and instead I was shallow breathing more quickly from my chest. Sometimes, I find myself holding my breath altogether during moments of stress or concentration.

Rebecca told me more about how we breathe and how the diaphragm works and explained how we can all better connect with it. 'The diaphragm is the main muscle of respiration. It is a dome-shaped sheet of muscle and tendon seated beneath your lungs that plays a vital role in the breathing process. As we breathe in, we should feel the belly expand slightly as the dome contracts and compresses the abdominal space. As we breathe out, both the ribcage and belly should contract.

'Take a moment to visualize where your diaphragm is in your body,' she recommends. 'The organs above the diaphragm need to be connected and in communication with the organs below it, so there are openings for blood vessels and nerves.'

becoming aware of your breath

This exercise helps us to learn breath awareness and to think more about how we breathe. 'It allows you to quieten the thoughts in your head and connect to the feelings in your body,' Rebecca says. 'You'll become aware of your external and internal environment and feel completely aware and present. Like any practice, the most challenging part of breathwork is just sitting down to do it. Starting small and simple is the key and if you practise every day, it will soon become a way of life.'

1. Bring your focus away from your mind and notice how your breath moves through your body. Let your mind follow the flow of your breath. Be aware, observe and feel. Witness your breath coming and going.

2. How do you feel right now? Ask yourself: Am I tired? Am I happy? Am I anxious? Am I relaxed? Is my mind full? Am I overthinking? Am I focused? Whether it's positive or negative – without judging or controlling – just accept those feelings.

3. Are you carrying any tension? Where does your body feel tight? Where does it feel more free? Start tuning in to your body. Become aware of physical sensations, notice the contact of your feet on the ground, your sitting bones on the chair or floor. Be aware of your spine – is it straight? Are you hunching?

4. Become more conscious of your inhale and exhale and notice each one. Can you focus on bringing in more breath in a relaxed, flowing motion, slowly breathing in through your nose and out through your nose? Notice how that feels.

5. As you breathe in and out, pay attention to whether your jaw is relaxed or if you are slightly clenching it. Relax your jaw, allow the bottom jaw to have space and drop your shoulders. Just by bringing your awareness to your breath, you can start to feel truly present and conscious of how you feel. You come out of the mind and into the body.

6. Continue taking slow, gentle breaths. Now, inhale for as long as you can and breathe out for as long as you can. When you breathe consciously, everything changes. When you breathe with awareness, all day, every day, there is a cumulative effect. Bringing full awareness to your breath moves you from doing to being. As you hit the pause button on your busy mind, notice how you begin to change your state of being.

7. Bring the movement of your breath down into your lower abdominals. See if you can move the belly as you breathe in and out. This is where you start to consciously breathe with intention.

8. Expand your breath into your lower belly as you inhale and notice how the belly contracts as you breathe out.

9. Now, breathe in for a count of three and breathe out for a count of three. Make these simple, easy breaths, in through the nose and out through the nose, with no force, pushing or trying to control the breath.

10. Keep practising this for a few more breaths, going at your own count and pace. Remain aware of your breath, observing how the inhale feels and the exhale feels. Is it easier to inhale than to exhale or the other way round? Or do both feel the same?

'Practise this every day,' Rebecca recommends. 'As your breath is moving in and out you are completely aware and present with your breath. Breath awareness helps you to quieten the thoughts in your head and connect to the feelings in your body. It allows you to become aware of your external and internal environment.'

REBECCA'S EXERCISE FOR

REBECCA'S EXERCISE FOR
deep diaphragmatic breathing

Rebecca told me an astonishing fact – that there is as much lymph fluid in the body as there is blood! 'The lymphatic system is part of the immune system protecting us from illness and infection and this fluid flows through a network of lymph nodes and vessels all over the body,' she explains. 'One of the important aspects of deep diaphragmatic breathing is that it is a primary way to stimulate the lymphatic system to work at its full pace. Sixty per cent of all lymph nodes are located just under the diaphragm – so this breathing exercise hugely supports the immune system. We often hold tension in the diaphragm, especially when trying to control pain or emotions. We need to work with our primary breathing muscles – the lower abdominal muscles and intercostal muscles – to achieve a good diaphragmatic breath.'

Rebecca showed me the following exercise to help to bring my awareness to my breathing and ground and focus my attention. 'Think of it as a mini-workout for the respiratory system,' she suggests, 'and practise it as many times as you like. Although this can be easy to achieve, it takes repetition for the muscles to remember that action and requires letting go of old patterns in order for it to become automatic. You can do this exercise sitting up anywhere – at your desk, on the train or at home on the sofa.'

Here's what to do:

1. Rest your hands on your lower belly so you can feel your breath expanding and moving through your body. When you breathe in, the diaphragm contracts and flattens downwards, creating a vacuum that draws in air. When you exhale, the diaphragm returns to its dome shape, pushing air out of your body.

2. Keep your spine long and feel your sitting bones on your seat and your feet flat on the ground. Hold your head in a neutral position as if there is a thread at the centre of the top of your head, holding it up towards the sky. Allow your jaw, throat and shoulders to relax.

3. Breathe in slowly through your nose. Allow the slow, gentle inhale to expand your belly, pushing it out. Expand your sides and lower ribs, filling the diaphragm, back and lower back. Now let the breath go. Exhale with a gentle sigh through the nose or mouth and feel the belly contracting.

4. Place your hands around the lower ribcage as if you are giving yourself a hug and breathe into this space. Let your belly expand as you inhale and contract as you exhale. Keep your shoulders and jaw relaxed.

5. Repeat 5 to 10 times with hands on the belly, then round the ribcage and notice how you feel. Present, grounded, sleepy, relaxed?

BELLY BREATHING

I found it hard to bring my breath down into my belly at first, so this is what Rebecca recommended I do. 'Lie face down on the floor and make a little pillow for your head with your hands. As you breathe, feel your belly pushing into the ground as you inhale and letting go as you exhale. Then see if you can get the breath movement to come down into the pelvis, the space in between the hips. Practise this for a few minutes every day. It will eventually help to bring the breath movement lower down and activate these primary breathing muscles.'

NOSE AND MOUTH BREATHING

Rebecca teaches some exercises with the mouth open and some breathing through the nose. She told me more about the difference. 'Your nose is the first line of defence before air reaches your lungs, The hairs, mucus and cilia in your nasal passages catch and dispose of irritants like dust, pollen and pollution. They also catch potentially infectious bacteria and viruses. Nitric oxide is produced in the nasal passages and sinuses and can kill bacteria, and the bitter taste receptor in your olfactory system also helps to trigger your body's immune response. It's basically your body's home security system. When you feel stressed, unwell or anxious, your breathing is affected and you might catch yourself sighing, clenching your jaw or mouth breathing.

'But breathing through the mouth is not bad all the time,' she clarifies. 'And it's often very necessary and natural. For example, it's essential and natural to breathe through the mouth during childbirth, or when you sing or laugh. As you speak, your mouth is open, taking in little sips of air. And when you exercise, you need more air, so the mouth instinctively opens. However, it has been shown that when runners train themselves to breathe only through their nose, they can actually increase their stamina and reduce fatigue.

'While mouth breathing can be used for more advanced breathing techniques, in everyday life it's advisable to breathe through your nose,' Rebecca recommends. 'If people want to breathe deeper or use the breath for therapeutic work, they often breathe through the mouth and despite some claims that this stimulates the fight-or-flight response, when using mouth breathing techniques with intention, people can go into a very deep state of relaxation. The more you play with it and explore breathing exercises, the more you become attuned to what techniques work for you.'

THE NERVOUS SYSTEM

It is useful to know a little about the nervous system when thinking about breath. The body's involuntary functions, such as heart rate, blood pressure, digestion and respiratory rate, are regulated by our nervous system. As Rebecca explains, 'The parasympathetic nervous system (PNS) works to calm us, allowing us to rest and digest. It slows the heart rate and lowers blood pressure and breathing rate, while diverting blood supply towards the digestive and reproductive systems.'

'The sympathetic nervous system (SNS) counteracts this – it gets us ready for fight-or-flight when under stress, raising the heart rate, blood pressure and breathing and diverting blood to our brain and muscles. Breathing exercises can be a way of helping us override the SNS. With them, we can interrupt the hormonal reactions that contribute to chronic stress levels and can predispose us to anxiety.'

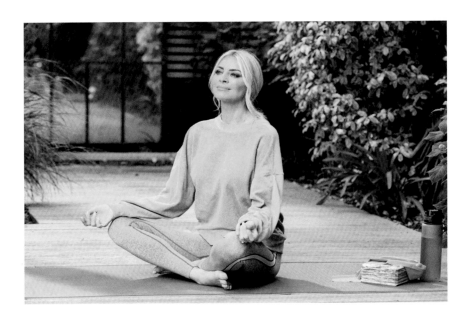

BREATH IS THE
BRIDGE LINKING
YOUR MIND, BODY
AND NERVOUS
SYSTEM.

learning to breathe

Despite the recent explosion of interest in wellness and an increasing appreciation of how important our natural health is, very few people are aware of the detrimental effects that improper breathing can have on their wellbeing. Something that Rebecca said really struck a chord with me. 'While most of us know instinctively how to breathe to survive, we aren't taught how to breathe to thrive. From your earliest childhood, you probably recall being told to "take a deep breath" when feeling upset, angry or anxious. Intuitively, we all understand, even if we've never heard the science, that how we breathe and how we feel are intrinsically linked.

take a deep
breath

'If you want to find a true breath guru, take a look at a sleeping baby,' Rebecca suggests. 'As babies and toddlers, we naturally breathe deeply from the diaphragm. We feel no inhibitions and have no awareness of feelings of fear, shame, guilt or embarrassment. We express exactly how we feel and are completely present. Our minds are not flitting all over the place and we are not trying to control our emotions or feelings by holding our breath or breathing shallowly to hide or not be heard.

'Between the ages of three and seven, we begin to develop emotionally, becoming more aware of our surroundings, culture and peer group, and of authority in the home and at school. In short, we become conditioned through being told to calm down, be quiet or brave. All these instructions create boundaries and obstacles when we are feeling emotions such as anger, embarrassment, frustration, sadness, guilt and joy – even when we are trying to stop ourselves from laughing. Dysfunctional breathing comes from learnt behaviour as well – children puff out their chests to look strong like superheroes; they're told to hold in their tummy in gymnastics and dance classes.'

Rebecca's advice is that to really harness the power of our breath, we don't need to learn new tricks, we just need to remember how we used to breathe.

I am already starting to find breathing properly makes a massive difference to how I feel during the day. I loved that during our work together, Rebecca told me to 'take my diaphragm to the gym' with breathing exercises. Now, I find myself practising them all the time. Here are just a few moments in everyday life that we can use for breathwork:

+   traffic jams

+   travelling to and from work on the train or bus

+   queueing at the supermarket

+   waiting for the kettle to boil

+   chopping vegetables for dinner

+   standing on the escalator

+   before going to sleep at night

Try to take some special moments, too. Set your phone to remind you a few times a day to take a break for 5 minutes and do some breathing. See what works for you. I'm still working on mastering this new/old art so that it becomes second nature – just as it was when I was a child.

REBECCA'S EXERCISE FOR

REBECCA'S EXERCISE FOR
expanding your breath

'You can do this exercise anywhere,' Rebecca says. 'It helps you to develop a better connection and understanding of your diaphragm and to use this primary breathing muscle more effectively.' Here's what she suggests you do:

1. Relax your shoulders – try not to hunch them – and close your eyes.

2. Inhale through the nose and exhale through the nose.

3. Repeat this 2 or 3 times, breathing in and breathing out.

4. Now wrap your hands around your lower ribcage. Bring the movement of your breath to your hands.

5. Breathe in through your nose and out through your nose. Visualize a triangle shape pointing down towards your pelvic region. Visualize your breath starting at the point of the triangle and expanding out into the ribs to fill the shape as you inhale, then contracting as you let go.

6. Notice where you can feel your breath and visualize the breath expanding in and out as opposed to up and down. Feel your breath moving your belly and ribcage as you keep your shoulders relaxed and your breath expansive.

discover your breath

In the West, we have been particularly guilty of ignoring the significance of breath, whereas it has been central in Eastern cultures for thousands of years. *Prana*, as it is known in India, or *qi* in China, means life force or energy and is the very essence of our being. The flow of *prana/qi* through the body is powered by the breath and is vital for both mental and physical health.

But Rebecca tells me that hardly anyone over three feet tall is truly breathing to their full capacity! That is astonishing. I very often find I'm holding my stomach in without meaning to – just habit, I guess, from years as a model – so I'm a chest breather. Allowing my stomach to relax and become part of the breathing process feels like a game-changer for me. It helps to calm me and focus my thoughts and energy – I love it.

BREATHING PATTERNS

Rebecca says, 'On high streets and school runs, in offices and homes everywhere, you'll find tight jaws, tight minds and tight bodies as we keep to tight schedules. There are a lot of different breathing patterns out there: we might be chest breathers, belly breathers, shallow breathers, frozen breathers, reverse breathers, breath holders and breath gaspers and so on. No two patterns are ever the same. Our breath mirrors our life patterns, yet some of these established patterns are not serving us well. The more you practise breathing well, the more you let go of any restricted breathing patterns and live life more freely.'

Chest breathing

'This is the most common pattern and it forms over time from holding the belly in to look thinner and as a response to stress. The movement of the breath is more in the upper chest. The shoulders rise on the inhale and there is a tendency to overuse muscles that you do not need for breathing. This can cause tension in the upper back and shoulders.'

Belly breathing

'In this, the movement of the breath is mostly in the belly but there is no or little movement in the ribs and chest area. The upper back can often feel tense. For a full open breath, the movement should begin in the belly and move up into the midsection, the ribcage and the chest.'

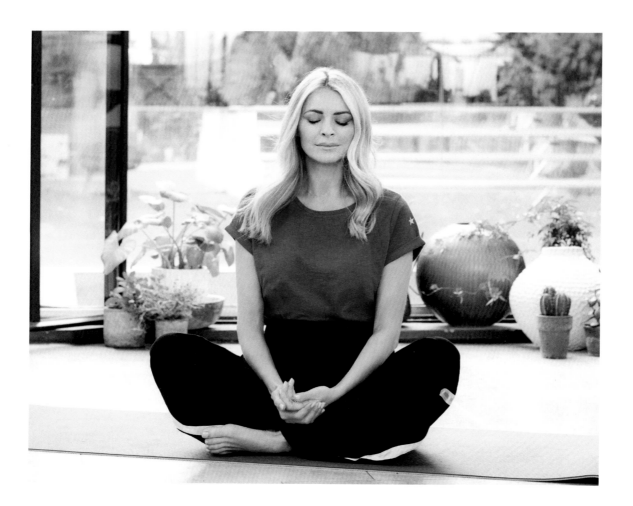

are you a belly breather or a chest breather?

Rebecca's simple exercise can help you begin to understand your breathing pattern:

1. Lie down or sit up, keeping your spine straight. Relax your shoulders; try not to hunch them. Close your eyes.

2. Take a breath in through the nose and breathe out through the nose.

3. Repeat this 2 or 3 times.

4. Now, place one hand on your belly and the other hand on your chest. Continue breathing in and out through the nose and notice where you feel the breath. Can you feel it more in your chest or in your belly or can you feel it equally in both? Wherever you feel your breath more indicates your dominant breathing pattern.

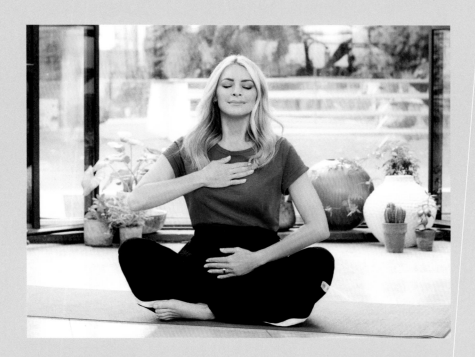

TAKING A MOMENT

Thanks to constant outside stimuli – our phones, for a start – our minds are busy racing, bouncing from one thought to the next. Our attention spans have certainly suffered as a result. Rebecca told me that 20 years ago, Microsoft measured the attention span of 3,000 adults in Canada and the average came in at just 15 seconds. In 2012, it was measured again and it had dropped to 8 seconds. Even a goldfish apparently has a 9 second attention span!

One of the reasons I really love to read is that it demands your full attention – you are in the moment and at one with that book, all outside distractions temporarily and luxuriously forgotten. I always feel so much calmer after losing myself in a good book. But it's not always possible to pick up a book. You may be in the middle of errands, a work meeting, making dinner or in a demanding situation that requires your full attention. For me, this is when conscious breathing – focusing on the breath with awareness – really comes into play.

Like meditation, conscious breathing helps focus thought and quieten the outside 'noise'. However, unlike meditation – which I admit to constantly trying to master but never quite nailing – it doesn't necessarily require you to sit quietly in solitude without distractions, trying to silence all thoughts. The benefits, however, are strikingly similar. I haven't thrown in the towel on meditation yet, but it is still a work in progress for me.

FOCUS

If, like me, you find it difficult to silence those thoughts entirely, then taking a moment to focus on your breath is a small step that could really make a big difference to your wellbeing. And yes, the whole quiet room/phone-off thing can help, but it isn't a necessity. I simply started on my own conscious breathwork journey by literally taking a deep breath. Then by counting while taking those breaths: in and out. The simple act of counting is often enough for me to centre and focus thoughts and stop my mind wandering.

LIKE MEDITATION, CONSCIOUS BREATHING HELPS FOCUS THOUGHT AND QUIETEN THE OUTSIDE 'NOISE'.

breathing through stress and tension

When did our lives become so busy? I'm sure I'm not alone when I say that I sometimes feel like I'm under constant bombardment from busyness and stress. I never seem to stop.

Modern life means we are all living with constantly busy schedules and it can sometimes feel like we're battling to keep burn-out at bay. But Rebecca's response is that feeling stressed isn't in itself a disorder – it's a response to the environment in which you put yourself and the barrage of information you take in from the outside world.

'A build-up of stress over time, though, is not good for you,' she warns. 'The maxim "Keep calm and carry on" might look great on a poster or a coffee mug, but it urges us to bottle up a maelstrom of emotions. Today's hamster wheel of inboxes, societal expectations, rolling news and sleep deprivation means that continuous low-level stress is now accepted as normal. But too much stress is damaging to our health.'

continuous low-level stress is now normal

FIGHT-OR-FLIGHT

Often, challenging situations, or even mundane events such as being late for a train, can put us into a stressed 'fight-or-flight' mode. Rebecca explains that our bodies are designed to maintain balance (the medical term is 'homeostasis'). 'But,' she says, 'we have not adapted and evolved fast enough to cope with being triggered constantly by the demands of modern life, so most of us are living in a state of constant low or high anxiety.

'This pressure triggers raised levels of the stress hormones cortisol and adrenaline, which lead to those all too familiar "fight-or-flight" feelings of increased anxiety. Stress can cause inflammation in the body; it messes with our minds and hampers our digestion. It won't allow us to rest easy or sleep adequately. And, of course, it also affects the way we breathe, causing us to take shorter, quicker, less efficient breaths, resulting in yet more problems in the body. Most of us have had moments of stress that have made us breathe faster, and in more extreme cases, this can become a panic attack.'

our emotions and breathing are fundamentally linked

Like so many of us, I'm guilty of clenching my jaw when feeling stressed or when concentrating, such as when driving, for example, or tapping away on a keyboard and looking at a screen. I don't even realize I'm doing it! I also get tight shoulders and pain around the neck, mostly as a result of not releasing this tension and instead holding on to it tight. Sometimes I also find myself holding my breath, without meaning to, and therefore just not breathing adequately or thoroughly enough. Rebecca says that constant tension in the body can also lead to:

+ anxious thought patterns

+ bad digestion

+ a weaker immune system

+ increased acidity and inflammation

It's all connected. Science is now catching up with what the sages and yogis have been saying for thousands of years: our emotions and breathing are fundamentally linked.

'When your fight-or-flight response is frequently triggered, which is common these days, you default to chest breathing and the breath can feel jerky, rapid, irregular or shallow,' Rebecca explains. 'Over time, if this becomes habitual, these muscles become overused and your breath becomes restricted to your chest. Since we have more blood capillaries in the lower lungs, upper chest breathing results in a less efficient oxygen exchange than deep diaphragmatic breathing. We don't take in as much oxygen with each breath and it's oxygen our body needs to regulate itself.'

DISCOVER YOUR DIAPHRAGM

'The breath is the bridge linking your mind and body and nervous system. It's possible,' Rebecca says, 'to change the messages being sent from the body's respiratory system to the brain by voluntarily changing the rate, depth and pattern of breathing.

'Breathing techniques provide a portal to the autonomic communication network, enabling us to make a change in our breathing patterns. We can send specific messages to the brain using the language of the body, a language the brain understands and responds to.

'The practice of diaphragmatic breathing helps to stimulate the parasympathetic nervous system (PNS), bringing us to a calm state and allowing the body to rest and digest. The expansion and contraction of the diaphragm when you breathe correctly through your nose can also stimulate your lymphatic system and act to "massage" your internal organs. The lymphatic system works with the immune system to help the body remove internal toxins, so you can start to understand how something as simple as breathing well can increase your body's natural detoxification process.'

releasing everyday stress

Rebecca has found that people who are overstressed or hovering in a state of low or high anxiety breathe more in their upper chest than into the belly. If you are finding it impossible to get any movement in the belly when you breathe, try this:

1. Lie down on your back with your knees bent and feet flat on the floor. Allow your arms to rest by your sides and have a sandbag close by. (If you don't have a sandbag to hand, a bag of rice or a heavy book will do.)

2. Establish a flow of relaxed breathing – feel your breath flowing in and out through your nose.

3. Bring your focus to your lower belly. Feel it rise as you inhale and fall as you exhale.

4. Let the breath flow with a little pause between the breaths.

5. Place your sandbag or book on your abdomen. Keep your hands on top of the weight so you can feel it moving. Simply placing the weight on the abdomen focuses your attention there. As you breathe, the diaphragm will rise as you inhale and lower as you exhale. Try to keep your breath out about the same length as your breath in. This not only strengthens the diaphragm but also tones the muscles of the abdomen.

6. Don't force the breath. Simply allow air to flow in and out of your body. Repeat this for a few minutes and notice how you feel.

'By releasing tension in this way, you can increase your lung capacity and boost the lymphatic system, helping detoxify and protect your body from bacteria and other threats to your health. Breathing deeply allows the diaphragm to drop downwards and the ribcage to expand, increasing oxygen flow in the body and helping to slow your heart rate, promoting feelings of calmness and relaxation.'

releasing neck and shoulder tension

I so often feel tightness around my shoulders and neck and find myself holding my shoulders up to my ears. Rebecca explained to me that we accumulate a lot of tension in the shoulders by repeatedly overusing the shoulder, chest and neck muscles, muscles that are not part of the primary breathing system but, over time, are conditioned to move with the breath. She showed me how to counteract this. 'There are two ways of breathing – horizontal and vertical,' she says. 'The difference between the two is that the first is the way we were anatomically designed to breathe, while the other is how we've learnt to breathe over time. If you suffer from a lot of shoulder and neck pain that just won't go away, then vertical breathing is likely contributing to your discomfort. Vertical breathing puts unnecessary strain on the shoulders and neck muscles from overuse. This paired with a more sedentary lifestyle working for long hours at a desk is not a good combination.'

1. Take a deep breath right now and notice how your breath moves. Do your chest and shoulders rise? Is the breath movement up and down? You may find that when you take a deep breath in, your shoulders rise towards your ears and the breath puffs out of your chest with not much movement in the belly area. You may feel movement in the mid-section but a tightness in the chest and less movement in the lower abdominals. This is known as clavicular or vertical breathing.

2. If you feel like your breath is moving up and down and you can feel your chest and shoulder muscles rising, try to retrain them. Rather than your breath rising up and down, feel your breath moving in and out, expanding the belly, lower back and the ribcage on the inhale and contracting as you exhale. Try to practise a more expansive horizontal breath – think of your breath expanding in and out like an accordion.

breathing through the day

Rebecca has shown me a number of exercises to help me connect with, and use, my breath throughout the day to improve how I feel from the moment I wake up to winding down to sleep at night. I would like to share them, in her words, with you, and I know you will find them as rewarding as I have.

'Conscious breathing is the foundation of breathing well,' she says. 'It can help you to develop an intimate relationship with your breath, so you can sense when it feels right or when it feels jerky, rapid and restricted; whether it's more difficult to inhale or exhale, or both.

'You can bring back clarity and calm to the body by intentionally manipulating the rate, depth, rhythm and pattern of your breath to send information to your brain. Breathing is an unconscious instinct but when applying conscious intention we can achieve profound results. Breathwork is both a science and an art.

'Remember to think of the way babies and toddlers breathe. They have no inhibitions or concerns about what other people think. Their brains are not yet conditioned to respond to fear and they breathe fully and freely; not holding their breath or causing tension by contracting the respiratory muscles.'

Tip

The inhale and exhale don't need to be a particular length; nor do you need to observe the ratio between the inhale and exhale. Make sure that the inhale and exhale are deep and full and practised without struggle.

waking up and grounding yourself

This exercise relaxes the muscles, calms the mind, promotes circulation and creates a sense of peace. It's an effective way to ground yourself and check how you are feeling at the start of the day. It promotes mental stillness while encouraging a deeper, more mindful breath.

Do this sitting down or lying in bed in the morning as you wake up and connect to how you're feeling at the beginning of the day. You can also practise this exercise at work, when you're on your phone, when someone is speaking or while studying to recharge and help you find fresh energy, or to help you sleep.

Like any practice, the most challenging part of this exercise is to make the time to do it.

Start small and simple by doing 5 rounds:

1. Lie down or sit comfortably in an upright position and close your eyes.

2. Take a very slow, long breath in through both nostrils for as long as is comfortable.

3. Relax your shoulders and encourage your breath to move to your lower abdominals and ribcage. Relax your jaw.

4. Hold the breath for as long as is comfortable – at no point should this feel hard. As you are holding your breath, relax your jaw, throat, neck, shoulders, diaphragm and abdominal muscles. The more relaxed you are, the easier it will be to hold the breath for longer.

5. Exhale through both nostrils for as long as is comfortable.

6. Repeat 5 rounds of this exercise and then pause and observe how you feel. As it gets easier, add on a few rounds and begin to build a broader and more expansive breath. Notice where you feel more space, more length and more strength, and acknowledge where you feel more energy and alertness.

'Espresso' breathing to fix that 4 p.m. slump

This technique is known as 'breath of fire' or kapalbhati breathing. 'This is a great way to boost your energy levels and the digestive system, especially if you are feeling sluggish or are experiencing that mid-afternoon slump,' Rebecca recommends. 'Before reaching for a coffee or sugar rush to get you through the afternoon, try this dynamic abdominal breath exercise to wake up the mind and get the digestive system moving. Be warned that this exercise can make you feel dizzy, so do it sitting down and if it feels too much, simply bring your breathing back to its normal rhythm. Go at your own pace.'

1. Begin by sitting in an upright position with your spine straight and your hands relaxed on your thighs.

2. Take a long, slow breath in through your nose. Then, pulling your tummy in, make a forceful breath out.

3. Your body will naturally inhale again, so focus mainly on your forceful exhalations as you continue this breathing technique. As you exhale your tummy comes in.

4. Start with a round of 10 and then take a long inhale and let go with a big sigh. Repeat for a round of 10 and then take a long inhale and let go with a big sigh.

5. Do this 2 or 3 times more and notice how you feel.

There are very few breathing techniques in which all of the air in the lungs is fully exchanged. Often (especially when we breathe inefficiently) some stale air will remain at the very bottom of the lungs. But the successive, rapid, forceful exhalations we do in this exercise provide a cleansing of the lungs. This creates a very slight carbon dioxide debt in your body, so that when you move on to practise a slower-breathing exercise, your breath is longer, deeper and it's easier to enter a calm and meditative state.

box breathing for an evening wind-down

'People with high-stress jobs, such as soldiers and police officers, often use box breathing when their bodies are in fight-or-flight mode,' Rebecca tells me. 'This technique is also relevant for anyone wishing to recentre themselves or improve their concentration. Box breathing is a simple way of returning your breathing to its normal rhythm and is also a great exercise to help you switch off from work and relax into the evening. It is easy to do, quick to learn, and can be a highly effective technique for people in stressful situations. Its aim is to clear your mind, relax the body and improve focus. When you feel you have no time or space, when you're looking after children, on the school run, facing tight deadlines, cooking or in the shower, this is a perfect go-to rescue remedy.'

1. Sit with your back supported in a comfortable chair and your feet on the floor.

2. Close your eyes. Breathe in through your nose while counting to 4 slowly. Feel the air enter your lungs.

3. Hold your breath while counting slowly to 4. Relax your shoulders and try not to clench your jaw. Relax into the hold and simply avoid inhaling or exhaling for 4 seconds.

4. Slowly breathe out for 4 seconds.

5. Repeat the inhale, hold and exhale at least 3 times. Ideally, repeat the three steps for 4 minutes, or until calm returns.

Tip

If you find the technique challenging to begin with, try counting to 3 instead of 4.

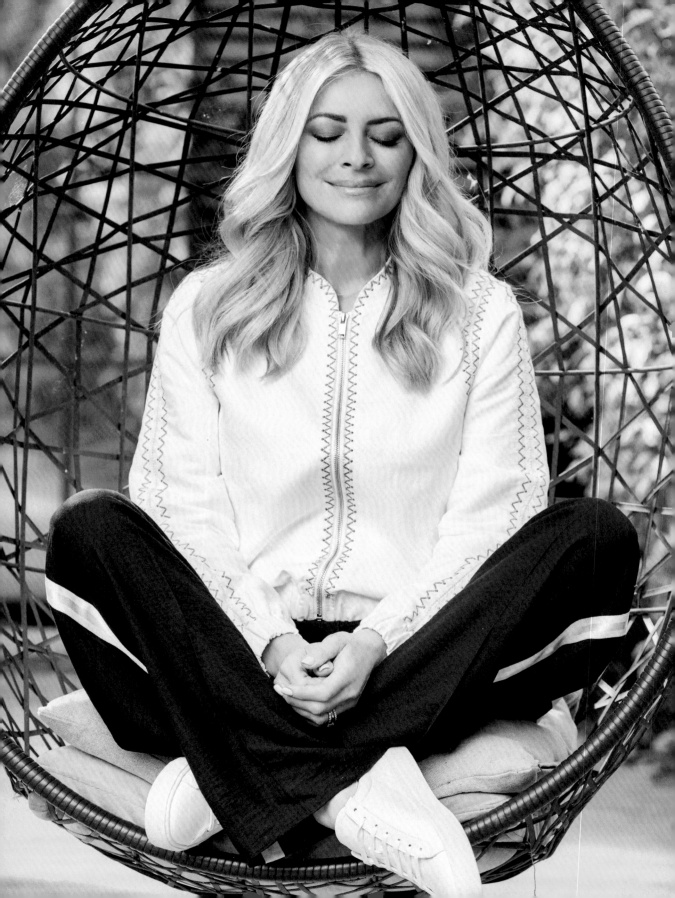

TAP INTO THE BENEFITS OF BREATHING

- Breath is life force. Breath is vital for both our mental and physical health.

- Be conscious of your breathing. The simple act of focusing on your breath can actually help calm and focus the mind in an instant.

- Conscious breathing helps focus the mind. In our busy lives, as we are regularly bombarded with constant stimuli, it's important to take a moment to quieten the noise, and conscious breathing will help you do that.

- Emotions and breathing are fundamentally linked. Stress affects our breathing patterns, with shallow breathing reducing the amount of oxygen in each breath, yet breathing deeply reduces stress, which is well worth remembering in moments of need.

- Incorporate breathing exercises into your daily routine. None of these exercises takes long to do or requires any great effort or level of fitness, but they can dramatically improve your health and wellbeing if done regularly. Do them whenever you're sitting in a traffic jam or waiting for the kettle to boil or, most especially, before you go to sleep at night as part of your calming bedtime routine.

- Keep it simple. Try breathing like a sleeping baby who naturally breathes deeply from the diaphragm with no inhibitions or feelings of fear, shame, guilt or embarrassment.

- Practice makes perfect. As you practice, day by day you will find the breathing exercises become second nature and you will truly find that you are, in Rebecca's words, breathing yourself better.

- Don't hold your breath, relax and B R E A T H E!

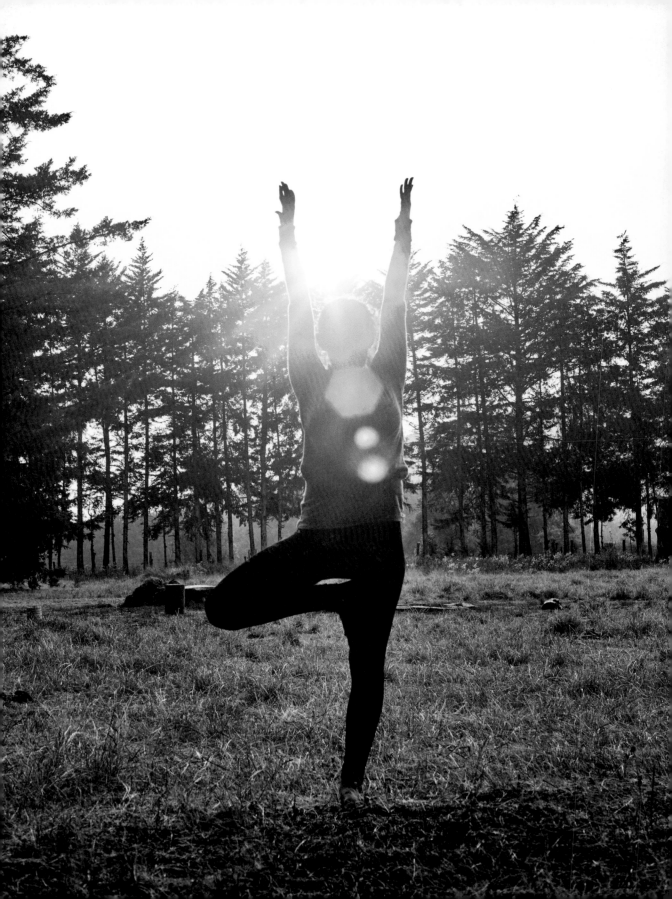

MOVE

Our bodies are
designed for
movement

simple regular activity

Our bodies are designed for movement – walking, running, stretching, bending – and being able to move around is something most of us take for granted. But modern life means that many people end up spending hours sitting at a desk, in the car or gazing at screens. I've read that health experts now say that sitting is the new smoking – that inactivity, particularly sitting for long periods, is seriously detrimental to our health.

sitting is the new smoking

Thankfully, simple regular activity really can make a huge difference, reducing the risk of illnesses such as heart disease, some types of cancer (including breast cancer), diabetes and even dementia. It keeps you flexible and improves your mood, so helps you enjoy life more! It's a win–win.

Now if like me you're not a fan of perspiring, I want to reassure you that being active doesn't necessarily mean spending endless hours in the gym or playing a sport. Part of it is about just keeping moving, whether walking the dog, going for a run, cleaning the house, digging the garden, dancing in the kitchen or doing some exercise routines at home. Anything that's not just sitting on your bottom.

ACTIVE OR JUST BUSY?

I've always been someone who's constantly on the go and can't sit still for long, but I used to confuse being busy with proper exercise. I fooled myself into thinking that just because I was always running around working, picking up after the family, making meals and so on, I didn't need to exercise. I thought being busy meant I was moving enough and besides, I couldn't fit anything else into my packed days.

But now I know better. After some episodes of hip pain, which I put down to six consecutive years of carrying and balancing babies on those hips, I realized I needed to strengthen my body. I started working out properly – going to the gym and doing some stretches and exercises at home as well to improve my strength and flexibility. I now appreciate how much it has helped me to have that investment of time in myself. Like many women, as a nurturer and caregiver I tended to put other people's needs first and my own last – sometimes to the point of near burnout. That had to change. When I exercise, I'm better tempered and more patient with the children and those around me. If I take that bit of time to care for myself, I feel better equipped to care for everyone else too, so we all benefit.

I really wasn't a gym bunny when I was younger but now I love my workouts and I do a couple of sessions a week. That way it's fixed in my diary, and I'm less likely to make some lame excuse to get out of it or find something else that demands my attention. I usually work out with my great friend Sam, who also happens to be a brilliant personal

KEEP MOVING

I had a great example of the value of staying active when I first started working on *Strictly* back in 2004. The late, great Bruce Forsyth was an inspiration. He was well into his seventies then but always seemed to have boundless energy. He would literally leap up from his seat to standing and was full of beans, raring to go even after a 12-hour studio day. Also, he had the best posture of us all, never stooped or hunched. And even when he was standing talking to you, he'd be working a little tap dance with his feet. He'd be moving all the time – he didn't much like keeping still, did Brucie! In the 10 years I worked with him, I never once heard him complain about an ache or a pain. He credited the secret of his energy to a daily 30-minute exercise routine, practised by Tibetan monks, which involved lots of stretching and yoga-like movements that kept him flexible and fit. It certainly worked for him – he was 86 years old when he finally retired from *Strictly*.
What an amazing man he was.

trainer. He has helped me turn my own fitness around with his can-do, positive attitude and easy-to-follow but effective training routines. He kept me going during lockdown via Zoom sessions and I always felt so much better for having done them afterwards.

JUST TURNING UP!

For me, it's about staying strong and flexible without becoming obsessive. And while it may sometimes feel hard to fit in the exercise I know I need, I have found that it gives me strength – both literally and figuratively – making it easier to cope with the day-to-day demands of family life. Sometimes I might not feel like going for an exercise session and I arrive moaning and groaning, but afterwards I feel so good. I thank Sam for his unfailing patience and positivity when faced with my reluctance, and I leave with a big smile on my face. I've learnt that turning up is key and I've never yet regretted a workout!

Since having a more regular routine, my fitness has improved so much. I fly up the stairs rather than walk and I feel more able to manage everything else in my life. I don't get so tired. Exercise helps me mentally, because if you're strong physically you feel stronger mentally too – the two go hand in hand. I guarantee that you will feel much more positive after some physical exercise and that feeling makes the effort all worthwhile.

THE BENEFITS OF MOVEMENT

There's now lots of research on the effects of exercise, showing that activity is important in so many ways. Exercise boosts your circulation, pumping more blood around the body, improves the efficiency of the digestive system – which was news to me – and helps balance the bacteria in your gut. I've discovered that it supports the production of collagen, helping to keep your skin firm and maintain elasticity, so it makes you look better too. It even improves your sleep – exercise promotes the production of melatonin, which aids sleep. And exercise not only improves your muscle strength but also keeps your bones healthy, guarding against osteoporosis and possible broken bones in later life.

I'VE LEARNT THAT TURNING UP IS KEY AND I'VE NEVER YET REGRETTED A WORKOUT!

just get
moving in
a way that
suits you

I know we all feel that there just aren't enough hours in a day to cope with all the demands on our time, but my experience is that it really is worth finding something you like doing and sticking with it. It doesn't have to be complicated; you don't have to spend money on fancy kit, just get moving in a way that suits you. As soon as you start moving more, you'll feel more energetic and want to increase your activity levels – it's a virtuous circle, which makes incorporating exercise into your life easier the more you do it.

REPLENISH

We're taking from our bodies all the time and we need to give back with good nutrition, maybe some massage (even self-massage helps), quality sleep – and movement. Our bodies will thank us for it. And don't forget to keep your fluid intake up. If you're dehydrated, you won't perform as well. Drinking plenty of water – for females about 1.5 litres (2½ pints) a day and for males 2 litres (3½ pints) – not only keeps our systems working better but hydrates the skin too, giving us a healthy glow.

FIND SOMETHING YOU ENJOY

General guidelines on the amount of exercise we need suggest a minimum of 150 minutes of moderately intense exercise every week for cardiovascular health – that's activities such as jogging or running, walking briskly, cycling, dancing or playing a sport, plus a couple of sessions a week of exercises for flexibility and strength, such as yoga or Pilates or working with a resistance band. You may like going to the gym or exercising outdoors or at home. Try different things and see what suits you. Join a Zumba class, try some online classes as a taster, or just get out there and walk at a good, brisk pace – you'll soon feel the benefits.

More and more, we're learning that if we don't do any exercise at all, not only do our bodies get stiff and inflexible, our muscles weak and our bones more fragile, but we also run an increased risk of serious illness. It's important but let's make it fun too, because, as we all know, if we don't enjoy what we do, we just won't stick with it.

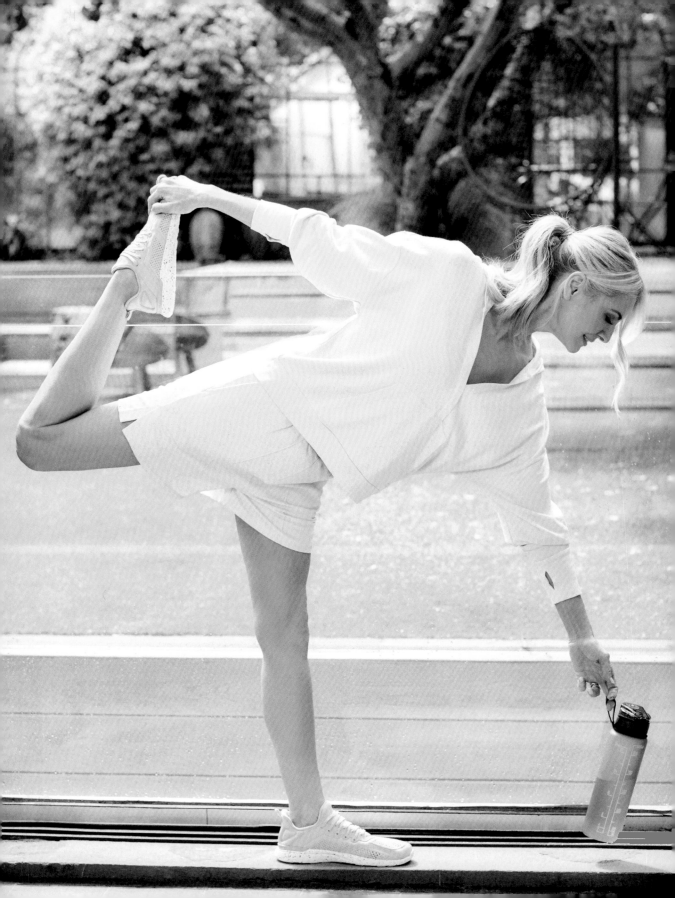

EXERCISING AT HOME

It's great to work out at a gym if you have the opportunity to do so, but if not, find a space in your home and the time in your day to do some stretches and exercises there. Start gently as recommended overleaf, particularly if you have any health conditions or you haven't exercised for a while.

Since Sam has helped me so much with my own fitness journey, I wanted to share with you some of his knowledge and the workouts we do together, as well as the importance of engaging in different types of exercises – for flexibility, strength and cardiovascular health. We've come up with ideas to help you and me keep active, without the need for special clothes, equipment or gym memberships. These are simple exercises that you can do at home and are easy to fit into your daily routine, plus some quick fixes to energize you during your working day.

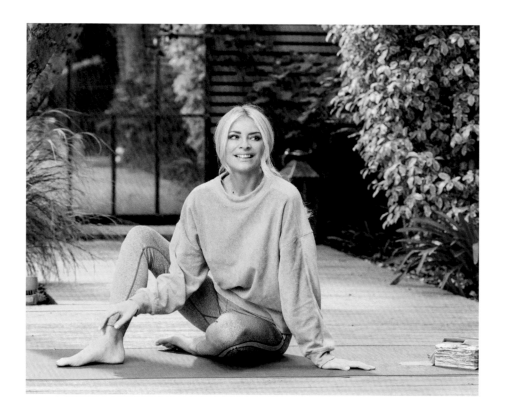

START GENTLY

If you haven't done any exercise for a while, be careful at first. And if you suffer from any health concerns or have had injuries, do check with your doctor or another health professional before starting.

A good way to ease into more activity is to start with a few brisk walks. Try for 30 minutes about 4 times a week and then step up your walking time and frequency. If your schedule allows, walk in the morning – it's good to start the day with movement and research shows that being out in the morning light helps us sleep well, too (more on this on page 228). Practise some of the exercises and stretches on the pages that follow and try to build more movement into your day, simply by standing up more and trying a bit of skipping or dancing. You'll soon find your enthusiasm growing and your fitness improving. And you'll discover that the more you do, the more you want to do.

When exercise becomes a habit, it becomes much less of a struggle and, believe me, it is so worthwhile.

CHOOSE A GOAL

Exercise isn't just about the body. It's also important for our mental health and wellbeing. By doing some form of daily exercise, you're not only building lean muscle, speeding up your metabolism and increasing your endurance, you're also improving your state of mind. When you exercise, your body releases hormones called endorphins, the feel-good hormones that trigger a positive feeling. I firmly believe that keeping fit and strong will help you cope better with the rollercoaster of life.

I hope I've encouraged you to get moving and gain the benefits of keeping your body moving. You might find it helpful to work towards a goal – perhaps a special occasion you want to look great for, or a charity walk or run you want to take part in. It helps to have an aim or a purpose and lots of people find that apps and step counters really increase motivation. Even a 10-minute walk helps.

quick fixes during the day

Even when you don't have time for a full workout, there are things you can do at odd moments during the day to help increase your activity levels and improve your fitness. Every minute counts.

Stand up

Just standing up instead of sitting down helps. Instead of slumping into a chair when you're on the phone, stand up – walk around too if you can. Simply standing up raises your heart rate, burns more calories and strengthens your bones.

To reset your body and get into a good standing position, squeeze your butt muscles and put your hands behind your back with your fingers interlocked. Engage your abdominal muscles and keep your hips in line. The more you do this, the more it becomes part of the body's muscle memory and improves your posture.

Walk on the spot

Try walking on the spot – even a few minutes at appropriate moments throughout the day is good and you can do it anywhere. Pump your arms as you do so. And once you get used to walking on the spot, you might even break into jogging on the spot.

Balance on one leg

This is something you can do while you're waiting for the kettle to boil, standing at the bus stop or even while cleaning your teeth. Don't worry if you wobble – everyone does at first – and wobbling shows there are brain and body connections going on and that's how you improve. If you practise every day, you'll soon get better at it. And once you can balance reasonably well on one leg, try doing it with your eyes closed, which is even more of a challenge.

Research shows that this simple act of standing on one leg is important not only for strength and balance but also for brain health, as it improves the coordination between your brain and your body. I set the timer on my phone and do 2 minutes on each leg, 2–3 times a day. I've found it really helps with pelvic and core stability. Most people find it harder to balance on one side than the other, so do extra practice on your weaker side.

Standing on a wobble board makes you work even harder and helps stabilize the core and strengthen the glutes – the muscles in your bottom. Wobble boards are available from gym equipment stores and online.

Challenge yourself even more by standing on one leg and throwing a ball against the wall, then catching it again as it bounces back. Your body will have to work even harder to maintain balance and coordinate your catching and throwing actions. It takes practice but as you improve, try throwing the ball higher or lower or off to the left and right.

Shaking

You'll often see athletes and sportspeople doing this before a race or a match. It's also something that's part of martial arts routines, such as qigong. Just stand with your knees slightly bent and start to shake your arms and your shoulders. Then gently bounce up and down into your heels, so your whole body is shaking. Keep your neck relaxed. Do this for a minute or two and you'll be warmed up and reinvigorated – a great wake-up routine on a cold morning!

Skipping

Skipping is cheap, simple, great for getting your heart pumping and you can do it anywhere. All you need is a bit of rope. I love to spend a few minutes in the morning skipping – particularly if I have to miss a gym session because of work. I'll time myself on my phone and do 1-minute skipping, 1-minute rest for 8–10 minutes. It wakes you up – even more than that morning cup of coffee, I promise you – and gets the heart rate up and those all-important endorphins kicking in. You'll be surprised.

Dancing

If you're feeling down and stressed, put some music on and dance for 5 minutes. It doesn't matter what you look like, you'll have fun, feel better and get your body moving. Swivel your hips and pretend you're on *Strictly*!

staying flexible

Flexibility exercises help to keep the joints moving and are increasingly important as you grow older to prevent stiffness and immobility. They include stretches, yoga, Pilates and tai chi. Doing these types of exercises 'oils' the joints and keeps them working effectively.

I also really enjoy yoga – more than the gym, to be honest, as there is much less sweat involved. It works wonders for my flexibility, helping to elongate and stretch any cramped muscles. Yoga also feels almost languorous to me – meditative if you like, especially once I get into the 'zone'. I tune out all the noisy distractions, turn off my phone, mute the doorbell and get into my head while doing the exercises. I find committing to the flow of the yoga poses and breathing consciously at the same time means that I feel fully present in the moment and my mind is calm and stilled.

I try to do an online class a few times a week and some stretches by myself every day. I find if I get up 15 minutes earlier and do my yoga, I really do feel so much better. It's not always easy, I admit, and some days I struggle, particularly in winter when the mornings are dark and cold and the alarm has gone off at 6 a.m., but it's worth it. It makes all the difference. Mostly, before I start, my head is telling me that I haven't got time to get online for 15 minutes and do a yoga workout, but every time I do it – without exception – I feel better as a result. The day seems to go more smoothly somehow, and I feel that even if it doesn't happen again all day – and it probably won't – I've had a few moments of me-time. I recommend you try it – you'll be glad you did!

some days I struggle but it's worth it

There are plenty of free yoga and Pilates sessions online but if you can, it is good to get to some classes and be face-to-face with a teacher in the room, particularly when you are starting out, so that you can learn the positions safely without doing yourself any damage.

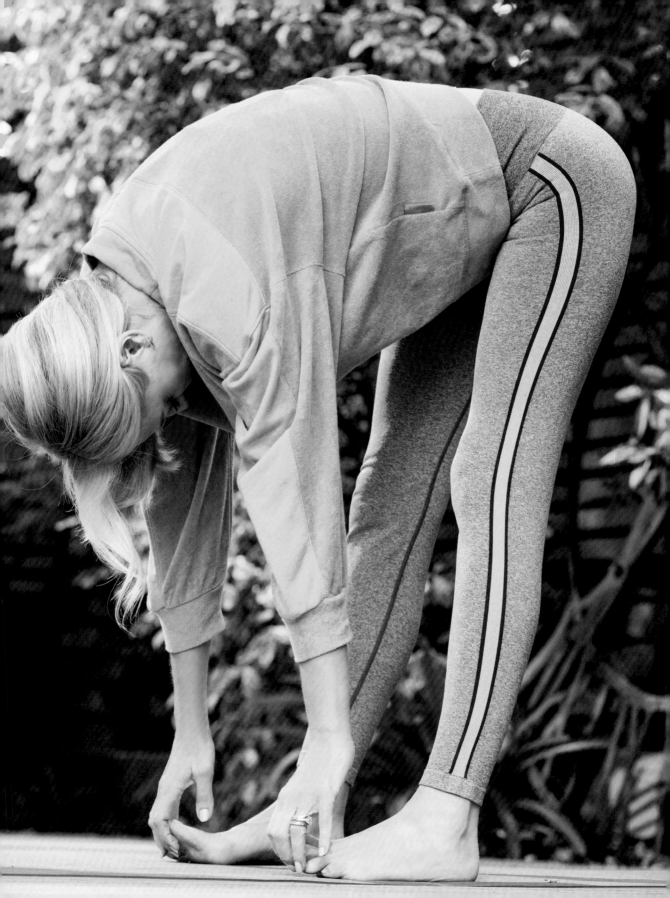

EXERCISE ISN'T JUST ABOUT THE BODY. IT'S ALSO IMPORTANT FOR OUR MENTAL HEALTH AND WELLBEING.

cardiovascular health

the good news is that you don't have to be a marathon runner to get these benefits

Exercise that raises your heart rate is very important. Running, brisk walking, cycling and cardio workouts get your heart and lungs working harder, sending extra oxygen and energy around the body. Your heart rate is the number of times your heart beats per minute. When you're active you need more energy, so your heart beats more quickly to enable it to pump enough blood to your muscles. As you exercise, your breathing deepens and quickens. An increased heart rate is a sign that you're training your body to absorb more oxygen and improve your cardiovascular fitness.

The heart is a muscle and giving it a workout by raising the heart rate strengthens it and makes it more efficient. Heart specialists say that the increase in blood circulation from exercise has many health benefits, including lowering your blood pressure and the risk of diabetes as well as reducing inflammation in the body. And the good news is that you don't have to be a marathon runner to get these benefits. Just aim to increase your heart rate for at least 30 minutes every day by doing something as simple as going for a brisk walk.

GUT HEALTH

The latest news is that cardio exercise improves gut health, so you're helping your body on all fronts. Research suggests that people with good cardio fitness also have a more diverse gut flora and that means a better balanced and healthier digestive system. For more about gut health in general, have a look at pages 16–50.

SAM'S EXERCISES FOR

dynamic warm-up stretches

Before you start doing a cardio routine or a run, it's important to warm up your body with some dynamic stretches – that means stretches combined with movement to increase the power of the stretch. These will also help maintain flexibility. Here are a few useful ones that you can do at home.

Walk outs

Mobilize your back, calves, glutes and hamstring muscles.

1. Stand with your feet hip-width apart. Bend forwards, hinging from your hips, and place your hands on the floor in front of your feet.

2. Shift your weight onto your hands. Start to walk your hands forwards until you are in plank position, with your hands on the ground beneath your head, legs straight and your back flat.

3. Then walk your hands back to your feet and stand up again. Repeat 6–8 times.

Hamstring sweeps

Great for stretching hamstrings and good for hip mobility.

1. Stand with your feet hip-width apart. Pushing your bottom back, place one leg straight out in front of you with your heel on the floor.

2. Sweep your hands forward over your feet and up towards the ceiling, then back down. Keep your back straight. Change to the other leg and do 10 sweeps on each leg.

World's greatest stretch

Great general stretch, which also works the pectoral muscles.

1. Stand with your feet hip-width apart. Bend forwards and place your hands on the floor, then walk your hands forward to a plank position. Keep your back and legs straight.

2. Bring your right leg forward next to your right hand. Lift your right hand and extend it, turning your body to the right.

3. Bring your right hand back down and through under the body to the left side, past the left arm. Repeat 6 times, then change to the other side.

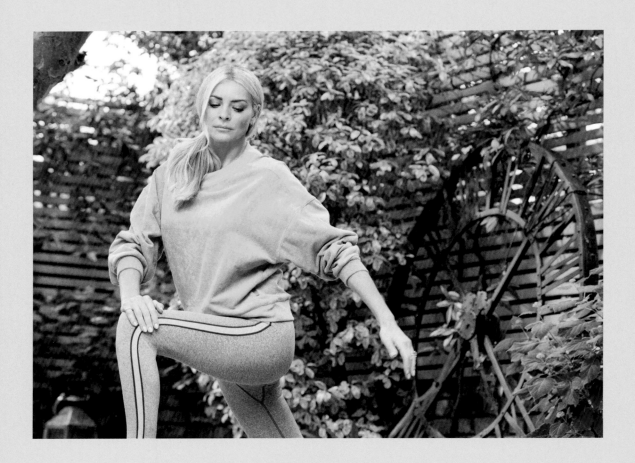

cardio activities

If you're into cycling or a particular sport such as tennis, rowing, football or whatever that's great, as you will get good exercise and have fun. I have to admit that I'm not that into sport, so my favourite ways of upping my heart rate are walking, skipping and swimming, as well as some of the cardio exercises described later in this chapter.

RUNNING AND BRISK WALKS

Some of my friends love running and it is a great way to exercise. You can do it anywhere, it's free and it's hugely beneficial. The NHS app Couch to 5k has had great success in getting beginners into running by taking things step-by-step and gradually building strength and stamina. You start gently by doing just 60 seconds of running followed by 90 seconds of walking and continue this for 20 minutes. You then build up week-by-week until you achieve that 5k goal. The app is free to download and contains all sorts of advice and tips to get you started and keep you motivated.

Personally, I'm not a fan of running, but that's just me. I worry that it puts a lot of stress on the hips and knees and it can make your face sag – trust me, at my age I don't want to accelerate that process! I prefer a brisk walk with the dog and recent research suggests walking at a decent pace is just as good for you as running. It can help heart health, reduces the risk of some types of cancers and of Alzheimer's in later life. And it's the easiest thing to build into your daily routine. It's important for your walking to be brisk in order to raise your heart rate. The British Heart Foundation's advice is that your walk should raise your heart rate and make you feel warm and slightly breathless. You

TRACK YOUR PROGRESS

I think we all find that it helps to have some sort of goal and there are various apps and devices to help you get the most from your walks. You can wear a fitness tracker to check your pace, distance, steps and so on, or simply download an app that checks you're walking at a good speed, not just ambling along. There is an NHS app called Active 10 that checks your speed and records your progress and this is free to download on your phone. The goal on the app is 150 minutes a week or just over 20 minutes a day, so start with that and build up to more if you can. If it's easier, you can break the total up into a few 10-minute walks a day at a pace fast enough to get your heart pumping. Or wear a simple step counter and aim for 7,000–10,000 steps a day.

should be able to talk but if you can sing, you're walking too slowly! You might also find it helpful to join in with other people. Check out the organization parkrun on the internet. They arrange 5k events every weekend in parks and other open spaces and it is free to join in. You can run, walk or jog – up to you. And there are 2k events for children, too. It's worth having a look to see what's happening near you.

SWIMMING

Swimming is a little harder to build into your weekly routine, but most of us have a public pool not too far away and there's always the increasingly popular wild swimming! Swimming is a great all-round exercise as it works the whole body and is good for the heart and for strength and flexibility. If you enjoy it, swimming is an excellent way of keeping fit and active. And take a tip from the Couch to 5k app – try doing a couple of lengths as fast as you can, then one or two more slowly. This will help to challenge the body and increase fitness and strength.

cardio fitness

These are all great moves to improve both your cardiovascular health and your muscle strength. They can be done at home with no special equipment.

High knees

A good warm-up exercise, this gets your heart pumping, strengthens your legs and improves flexibility.

1. Stand with your feet hip-width apart. Bring your right knee up towards your chest at a 90-degree angle, then lower it back down and bring your left knee up.

2. Continue alternating legs and pumping your arms at the same time. Go slowly at first if you are a beginner, then speed up as you get stronger.

Walking lunges

Good for working the muscles of the lower body as well as improving your balance. Obviously, it is useful to have plenty of space for this one, so you don't have to keep turning round. A good one to do in the park.

1. Stand with your feet hip-width apart, with your core engaged, chest up and shoulders back.

2. Take a big step forward with your right foot, keeping your weight in your heels.

3. Now bend your front knee and lower your back knee down to about 90 degrees. The back knee should lightly graze the floor.

4. Push through your right heel and rise to standing on that leg, as you drive your left leg forwards into a lunge.

5. Continue moving forwards with alternating lunges, remembering to keep your chest up and core engaged. If you don't have much space, turn as necessary.

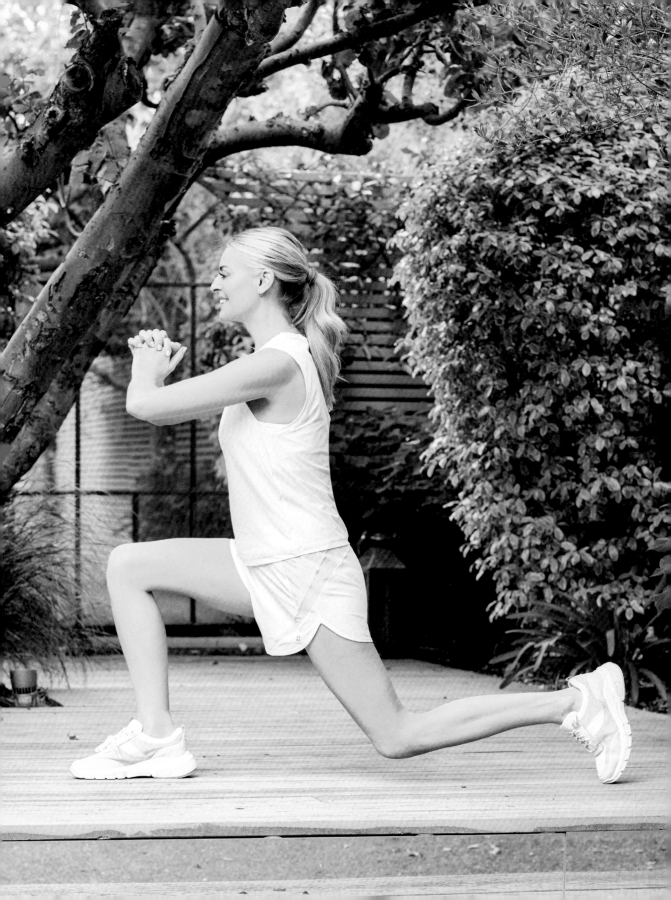

Body-weight triceps dip

Excellent for strengthening the arms and shoulders and an easy one to do anywhere you have a handy chair.

1. Sit on the edge of a chair. Hold on to the front of the chair seat with your hands, fingers pointing downwards. Keep your hands shoulder-width apart.

2. Place your feet out in front, keeping them together.

3. Keeping your back up against the chair, slowly bend your elbows to lower your bottom towards the floor.

4. Working your triceps, go past 90 degrees, then slowly push yourself back up, again focusing on your triceps.

5. Repeat 10 times.

Body-weight squats

Good for strengthening the leg muscles.

1. Stand with your feet shoulder-width apart. Keep your back straight, chest up and engage your core muscles.

2. Bending your knees, lower your bottom as though you're sitting on a chair.

3. Remember to keep your back straight and chest up and push your weight into your heels.

4. Keep lowering yourself down until your knees are at a 90-degree angle, then push back up, squeezing your glutes together. Use your abdominal muscles.

5. Repeat 10 times.

Half press-ups

Helps upper body strength and strengthens your core.

1. Position yourself on the floor in a half-plank – with hands and knees on the floor, toes tucked under. Start with your arms straight and keep your hands in line with your armpits.

2. Lower your chest towards the floor, keeping your spine straight and pushing your weight into your palms.

3. Push back up in a controlled movement, engaging your chest and core.

4. Repeat 10 times.

Half sit-ups

Great for abdominal strength.

1. Lie on your back on the floor – preferably on a mat for comfort. Have your knees bent and feet flat on the floor.

2. Put your hands out in front and engage your abdominal muscles. Lifting your head and shoulders off the floor, slide your hands up your thighs towards your knees – go as high as you can.

3. Slowly lower yourself back down, keeping your abs engaged throughout.

4. Repeat 10 times.

core
strength

One of the main aims of strength exercises is to strengthen your core – the muscles in your trunk that stabilize the spine, pelvis and shoulders. A strong core is all-important in preventing problems such as lower back pain. The core is the scaffolding of our body and everything benefits from it staying strong. If your core is weak, it affects everything else in the body.

If a muscle doesn't do much work, it gets weaker, so it's important to do some activities that make the muscles work a little harder than usual. These exercises increase your strength and help you carry out your daily tasks more efficiently. They also make it less likely that you will strain or injure yourself.

a weak core affects your whole body

Core-strengthening exercises involve using your body weight or working against resistance and include working with resistance bands, stair-climbing, push-ups and similar movements, yoga and Pilates. It is vital for improving overall muscle strength and also increases bone density, reducing the risk of bone diseases such as osteoporosis. After the age of about 35 to 40, our muscle power gradually starts to lessen, but regular strength training does help us to hold back the decline and maintain endurance.

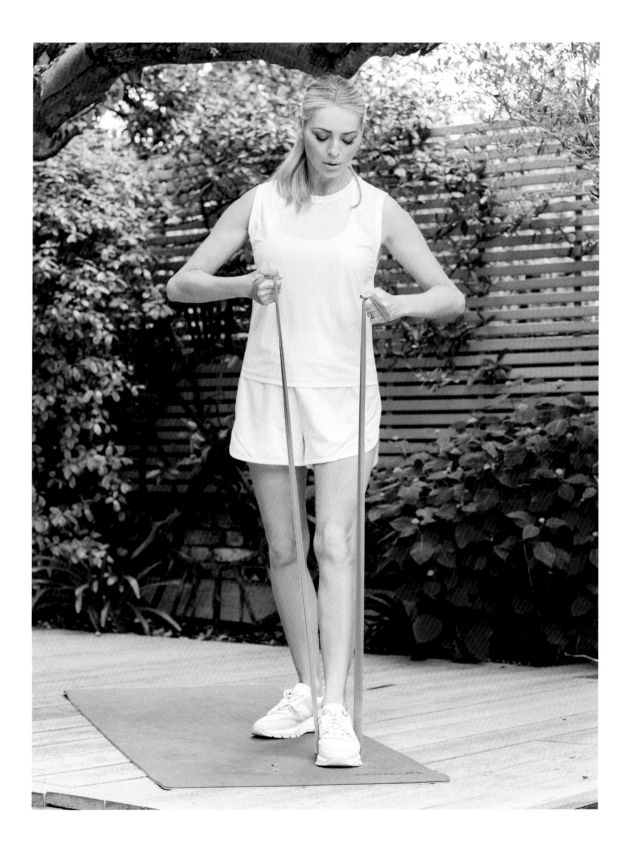

SAM'S EXERCISES FOR

core strength

The following exercises make a great core-strengthening routine. Do them gently and slowly at first and listen to your body. If something doesn't feel right, stop and check you're moving correctly. You'll find free instructional videos of all these exercises online, too.

Dead bug

Great for strengthening your lower back, abdominals and hips, while also improving coordination.

1. Lie on your back – on an exercise mat if you have one. Extend your arms straight up above your chest. Bend your knees and lift your feet off the ground so your knees are at a 90-degree angle. Remember to keep your lower back flat – don't let it arch.

2. While keeping your right leg and left arm still, reach your right arm back towards the floor while extending your left leg forward without allowing your foot to touch the ground. Bring your right arm and left leg back to the start positions and repeat with your left arm and right leg.

3. Repeat 10 times on each side, keeping your abdominal muscles engaged and your lower back pressed into the floor. Go slowly, making sure you keep breathing and checking that your pelvis doesn't rock back and forth. The more you can keep your core steady and stable, the more effective the exercise will be.

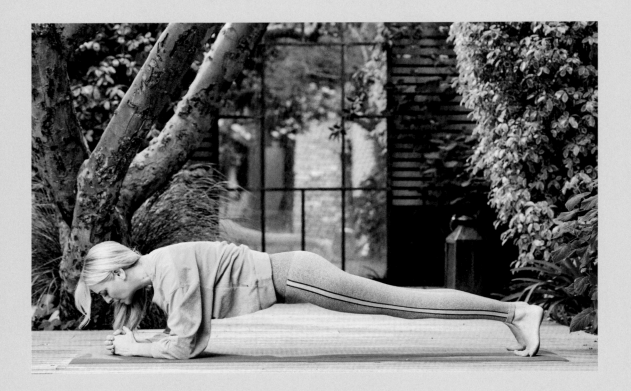

Plank

Good for strengthening your core and working the shoulders, arms, legs and glutes.

1. Lie on your tummy with your legs straight out behind you and elbows beneath your shoulders.

2. Tuck your toes under your feet and push your body up with your upper arms, leaving your forearms and hands on the floor, engaging your tummy muscles and squeezing your glutes. Remember not to let your lower back drop down or arch your back – you want your back to stay in a nice straight horizontal line. Look down at the floor between your hands and keep your shoulders level.

3. Remain in the plank position for 45–60 seconds, then gently lower yourself down. Repeat 3 or 4 times. If you can't stay in the position for long at first, gradually extend the time as you practise.

Slow mountain climbers

Strengthens the core while also improving hip and shoulder mobility.

1. Start in a plank position with your arms fully extended and locked straight under your shoulders, palms flat on the floor. Remember to keep your back straight – no sagging in the middle.

2. Keeping your tummy muscles engaged, tilt your pelvis inwards and bring one knee towards the inside of the elbow – or as close as you can make it. Do this in a nice, controlled manner and don't let your lower back drop.

3. Take the leg back and repeat with the other leg. Take it *slowly* – the slower you go, the more you work the core. Try for 14 repetitions, building up to 26.

Side plank

Works the oblique abdominal muscles and helps improve balance.

1. Lie on your right side with your legs straight out and in line with your hips. Your right elbow should be directly under your shoulder and your left arm along your left side.

2. Engage your tummy muscles and lift your hips and knees off the floor. Keep your body in a straight line – remember not to let yourself sag in the middle or your hips drop down towards the floor. Hold for 30–45 seconds, then carefully return to your starting position. Change sides and repeat. Do 3 or 4 repetitions on each side.

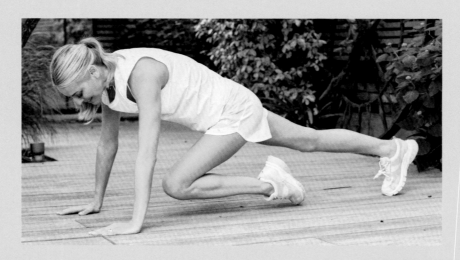

exercises with resistance bands

Stretchy rubber resistance bands are great for doing exercises that help improve core strength and are perfect for use at home. Some are like a loop while others are like a long ribbon. Both kinds are cheap, easily available online and come in different strengths. It's best to start with the lighter bands and work up to the tougher ones as you get stronger. They weigh next to nothing and take up very little space. Here are some ideas to start with and you'll find more routines online.

EXERCISES WITH A RIBBON BAND

These arm exercises are great for strengthening and firming your arms and increasing shoulder flexibility.

Bicep curl

Works the muscle at the front of the upper arm.

1. Stand up straight, shoulders down and collarbone wide. Move one foot slightly in front of the other and place it on the centre of your band. Hold one end of the band in each hand, with your arms straight down.

2. Keeping your elbows close to your sides, slowly bend one elbow to bring your hand up towards your armpit, then lower, feeling the tension from the band. Repeat with the other arm. Do 12–15 repetitions on each side.

3. Once you get stronger, try raising both arms at once. Again, do 12–15 repetitions.

Advanced (or wide-stance) bicep curl

Works the biceps a little harder.

1. Stand with both feet on the centre of the band, hip-width apart, which increases the tension on the band. Hold one end of the band in each hand, arms straight down. Shrug your shoulders up to mobilize them and release any tension. Repeat a few times.

2. Keeping your elbows close to your sides, bend your elbows to bring your hands to elbow level or all the way to your armpits.

3. As you get stronger, you can make the exercise harder by holding the band further down, which increases the tension on the band.

Triceps stretch

Works the muscle at the back of the upper arm – a great way to get rid of the dreaded bingo wings!

1. Stand on one end of the band. Hold the other end with one hand behind your head, elbow bent.

2. Looking straight ahead and keeping your spine still, straighten your arm up above your head to work the triceps muscle. Repeat 12–15 times, then repeat with your other arm.

Shoulders and lats (muscles in the upper back)

Works the upper back muscles, giving you a beautiful back for those summer dresses.

1. Stand with both feet on one end of the band, hip-width apart, holding the band on the right side of the body. Now transfer the band to your left hand, so it is going across the body.

2. Lift your left arm out to the side and up to shoulder height, keeping your pelvis steady and core strong. Don't allow the body to twist. Repeat 10–12 times.

3. Switch, so you are standing with both feet on the end of the band and holding it on the left side of the body. Transfer the band to your right hand, so it is going across the body, and lift your arm to shoulder height as before. Repeat 10–12 times.

Biceps curls with squats

Works the biceps and lower body.

1. Stand with both feet on the centre of the band, hip-width apart. Hold one end of the band in each hand, arms straight down.

2. Now bend your knees and squat as though sitting back on a chair, at the same time bending the elbows and lifting to elbow level.

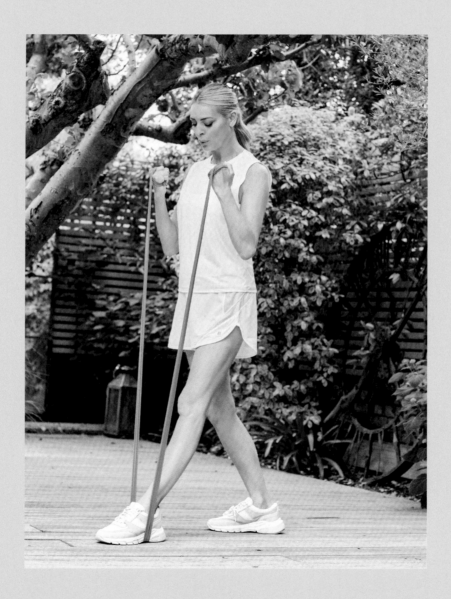

EXERCISES WITH A LOOP BAND

Great for isolating and working on particular muscle groups.

Shoulder muscles

Works your shoulder muscles.

1. Loop the band around your hands and hold your arms straight out in front of you at shoulder height, fingers pointing forwards. Keep your core strong and shoulders down.

2. Do 6 little pulses outwards, stretching the band.

3. Raise your arms straight up above your head. Relax your shoulders and pulse the band again for 6.

4. Lower the arms to shoulder height again and repeat. Keep going, alternating the movements for a couple of minutes.

Leg and hip muscles

Strengthens your leg and hip muscles.

1. Loop the band around your legs, just above the ankles.

2. Keeping your core strong and steady, lift your left leg out to the side, toes pointed. Lift and lower to a count of 6.

3. Now to work the quads, lift the leg to the front, toes pointed. Lift and lower to a count of 6. Remember to stay strong and stable.

4. For the glutes and hamstrings, move the left leg behind you and lift and lower for 6. Try to keep the spine still and don't let the body move forward and back.

5. Repeat all of the above with the right leg.

Sideways walk with a band

Works the glutes and hip muscles.

1. Place the band around your legs, just above your knees.

2. Stand with your feet shoulder-width apart, then bend your knees slightly and push them out wider than your feet. Keep your weight predominantly on your heels.

3. Keeping the tension in the band, slowly step sideways with the right foot. Don't let the band pull your knees in. Take 6 steps to the right, then 6 steps to the left. Keep going for 45 seconds.

Knee drops for hips and glutes

Great for strengthening your glutes.

1. Lie on your back with the loop band around your legs just above your bent knees. Keep your feet on the floor hip-width apart.

2. Drop your right knee out to the side, keeping your pelvis still, and bring it back. Drop the left knee out to the side and bring it back. Repeat 10 times on each side.

3. To make this a little harder, lift your hips up into bridge position and repeat the knee drops, then lower. Lift back up into bridge and pulse the legs out to a count of 10. Lower your back down, then repeat.

Side lifts for glutes and thighs

A good exercise for runners.

1. Put the loop around your legs above your knees.

2. Lie on your right side, with one arm stretched out beneath your head. You might like to have a folded towel between your head and arm to support your neck. Straighten out your legs in line with your spine.

3. Lift your left leg to hip height, then raise and lower 10 times.

4. Now lift your leg to hip height again and circle the leg 6 times in a clockwise direction, then 6 times anticlockwise.

5. Repeat, lying on your left side and lifting and circling the right leg.

cool down

At the end of an exercise session, a run or walk or class, it's important to help the body cool down with some stationary stretches.

Glutes stretch

The glutes are the muscles in your bottom. They're the biggest muscles in the body and help us with balance and every type of movement.

1. Lie on your back with your knees bent and your feet flat on the floor.

2. Lift your right leg to a 90-degree angle, then rotate it slightly and rest the right foot on the left knee and hold for 30 seconds.

3. Place your hands around your left thigh and lift the left foot off the floor to increase the stretch. If you find it hard to hold your thigh with your hands, you can use a stretchy band. Hold for 30 seconds, then release.

4. Repeat with the left leg.

Hamstring stretch

The hamstrings are the muscles at the back of the thigh, from the pelvis down to the knee. We use them all the time as we walk, run and move around and regular stretching helps improve flexibility and avoid injury.

1. Lie on the floor with your legs stretched out.

2. Put a towel or a resistance band around your right foot. Bend your left knee in and lift your right leg up. Hold it as straight as you can, without arching your back. Hold the position while flexing and straightening your foot.

3. Lower your right leg. Transfer your towel or band to your left foot, bend your right knee in and lift your left leg. Hold while flexing and straightening your foot as before.

Calf stretch

Another important stretch for keeping us moving well. Tight calves affect the movement of the feet and can cause injury.

1. Stand on a step. Keep the ball of the foot on the step and move the heel of your right foot back to rest off the back of the step.

2. Lower the heel down as you bend your left knee slightly. You should feel a stretch in the calf. Hold for 30 seconds. Repeat 2 or 3 times.

3. Change to rest the heel of your left foot off the step. Lower that heel as you bend your right knee and hold as before.

Cat-camel stretch

This is a good general stretch and great if you feel stiff after sitting at a desk for hours.

1. Get down on your hands and knees, with your knees under your hips and your hands under your shoulders. Keep your back flat – imagine you're balancing a cup of tea on it! Keep your abs engaged.

2. Let your head drop forwards and round your back up as far as you can so you feel a good stretch. Hold for 6–10 seconds, then return to your starting position.

3. Now lift your head up, let your back sink down and lift your hips. Repeat 6–10 times.

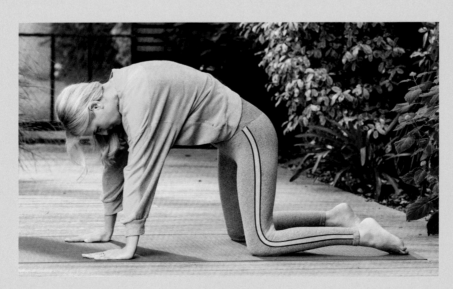

working day hacks

There are so many simple ways of building exercise into your daily routine without needing to set aside dedicated time or buy expensive kit. Just try walking at every opportunity, or doing a stretch or squat or two when reaching for something in the cupboard. Here are some of my top tips for incorporating movement into your day. I promise that once you start regularly doing just a few of these, you'll soon feel healthier and happier.

- Try to walk part of your journey to and from work. Maybe get off the bus a stop earlier or find a route that incorporates some opportunity to walk or cycle.

- Take the stairs rather than lifts or an escalator. I know – you've heard this a million times, but it really is worth doing. It increases your heart rate and strengthens your legs.

- If you have to spend most of your day at a desk, get up every half an hour or so for 5 minutes and have a quick walk around. Set a regular reminder on your phone and go and talk to a colleague instead of emailing or texting or simply walk up and down the corridor. If you work in a big building, try walking up the stairs to the next floor several times a day.

- When you're on the phone, stand up while you talk. Walk around as well if you can and roll your shoulders forwards and back a few times.

- If you have to meet with a couple of colleagues, how about trying a walking meeting instead of sitting around a table?

- As you sit in your chair, march your feet up and down as though you're walking on the spot.

- Stand up and hold on to your chair if you need support. Raise your heels off the floor so you are standing on the balls of your feet. Slowly lower your heels back down. Repeat 10–20 times and once you get stronger, do it without the support of the chair.

- Strengthen your all-important quad muscles by standing up from your chair – without using your hands. Keep your arms crossed across your chest and stand up straight. Slowly sit back down. See how many times you can do it in a minute, then try to beat your total next time.

- When you're waiting for the kettle to boil, do some counter press-ups. Put your hands on the kitchen counter, a shoulder-width and a half apart. Stand far enough back so that your arms are straight. With your body in a straight line, bend your elbows and slowly lower your chest to the counter, engaging your chest muscles. Push back up to straighten your arms again. Repeat 8–12 times, keeping your movements slow and controlled.

- If you like watching television in the evening, walk around the room at the end of your favourite show or during the commercial breaks.

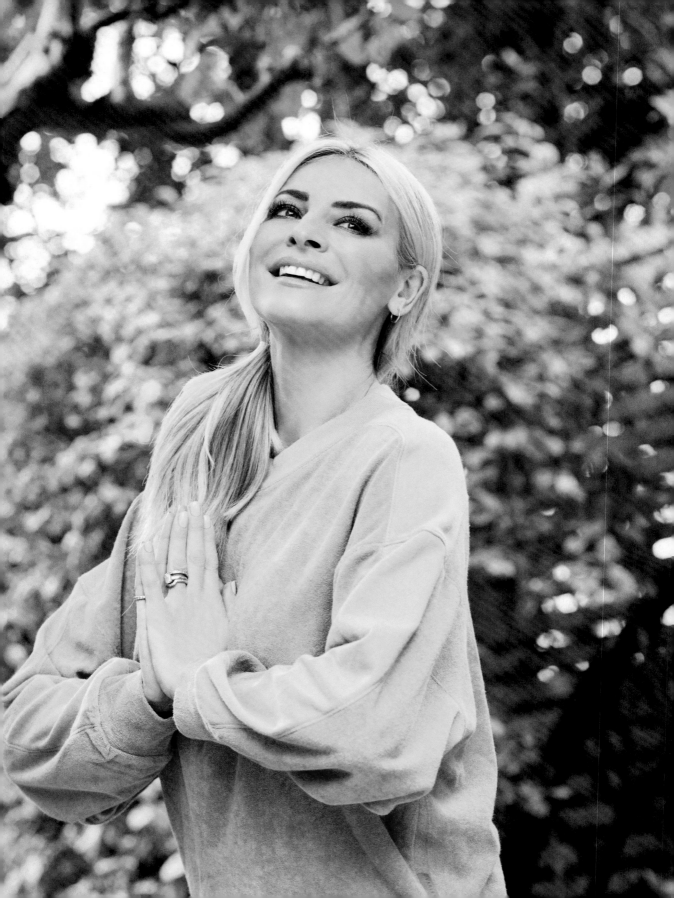

EXERCISE BENEFITS EVERY PART OF YOUR BODY, MIND AND SPIRIT

Exercise...

- lowers the risk of heart disease, stroke and diabetes, as well as some types of cancer.

- helps you lose weight and maintain a good weight.

- improves the body's ability to break down body fat and excess fat in the blood, so reducing the chance of obesity and metabolic disease.

- keeps bones and muscles healthy and reduces the risk of osteoporosis.

- aids sleep and gut health.

- improves your mood.

Aim to...

- do at least 30 minutes of moderate activity, such as brisk walking, 5 days a week, plus a couple of sessions of exercises to improve strength and flexibility. Remember to warm up and cool down after exercise sessions.

- reduce the time you spend sitting. Set an alarm or your phone to remind you to get up and move at least every hour.

- check with your GP before starting if you have health problems or if you haven't exercised for a long time.

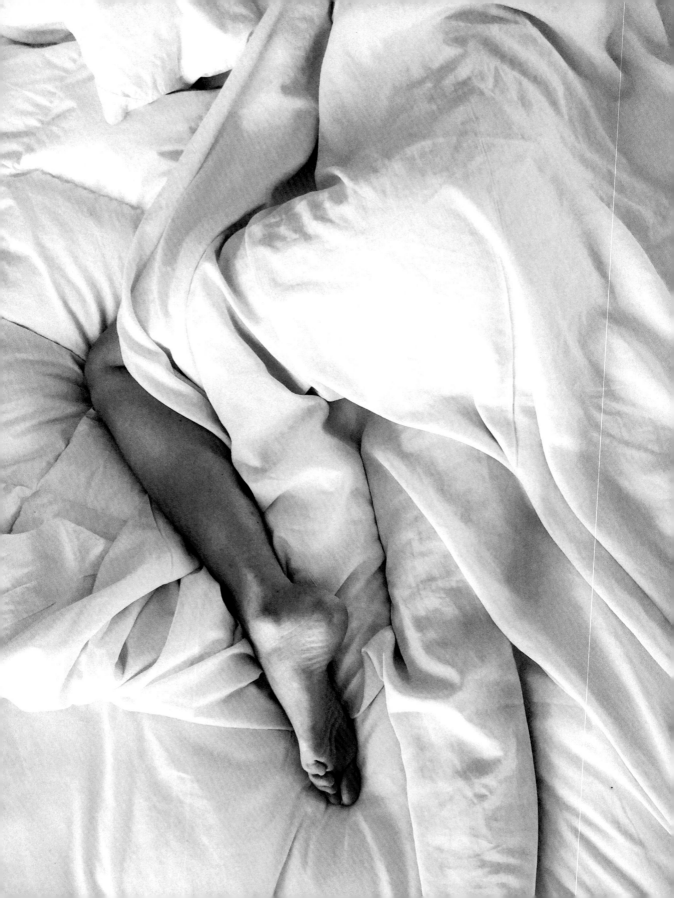

SLEEP

It's all about balance
... and habits

sleep is vital

Our fast-paced lives make it all too tempting to skimp on sleep. As a young adult, I tended to think of sleep as a bit of an inconvenience since there always seemed to be something better and more exciting to do – and so much to do, come to that. You can sleep when you're dead, I'd say to myself, so I'd go to bed late because I was busy and then get up early because I couldn't wait to seize the day! I was a night owl and a lark!

sleep is as important as eating well and taking exercise

But when I became a parent and went through repeated episodes of broken sleep with a baby demanding three or four feeds a night, I felt exhaustion beyond anything I'd known before: sheer on-my-knees exhaustion. Despite being in a new mum love bubble with my adorable baby, my sense of wellbeing would plummet after sleepless nights. I could barely think straight, such was my fatigue, and I realized I just could not function on a severe lack of sleep. My skin was dull and lacklustre and my usual happy-go-lucky mood was gone. And I seemed to get more colds because my immune system was obviously lowered by the lack of sleep.

I remember at that time being on *Strictly* and feeling so tired that I had to lie down on the sofa in my dressing room and close my eyes for 10 minutes. The next thing I knew, somebody was banging on the door and it was time for me to go to the studio floor. I'll never forget how I felt that day – I was so tired I could not physically get up from the sofa to walk to the dressing room door. I remember having to throw myself off the sofa onto the floor and literally crawl on my hands and knees the short distance to the door before dragging myself up with the handle. It sounds crazy now, but at the time it was sleep deprivation at its most torturous. I had to find the energy to get out there and work because, as they say in showbiz, the show must go on!

Living without a full night's sleep for over three years and having to work through it was downright traumatizing. I just couldn't go back to that dark place of sleeplessness! So, as a working mum, sleep became a priority. I began to understand just how vital sleep is and I realized that without it, I couldn't pull off either job effectively. When you think about it, we spend about a third of our lives asleep, which must show how totally crucial it is to our health – certainly not a waste of time. After all, sleep deprivation is a form of torture.

There's a huge amount of research now about the importance of sleep and what happens to our bodies while we sleep, and I've been finding out more with the help of Dr Linia Patel, who has shared her knowledge with me for this chapter.

SLEEP – A FOUNDATION OF WELLBEING

Linia is a very experienced dietitian and has spent much of her career helping athletes and other sportspeople achieve their best via nutrition. She explained to me that when you work with an athlete you're part of a team of trainers, psychologists and other experts, all of whom are dedicated to getting that person in the best possible shape, both mentally and physically. She then also became more involved in public health and in working with corporations, seeing clients such as bankers, lawyers and other high-flying execs. It was through dealing with them that she became fascinated with the whole business of sleep.

These people had high-pressure careers and worked long, demanding hours. Most prided themselves on being in the office early and staying late into the night. They often had to make long-haul flights across time zones and deal with jet lag. Their lives were all about proving they were the best; the hardest workers. And on top of all that, they would get up at the crack of dawn to do a run or workout to make sure they stayed fit. Very impressive, of course. On the face of it, these clients were doing everything right – eating well and exercising regularly – but they still weren't in the best of health. Linia found that her usual nutritional strategies weren't working, and these clients were showing signs of inflammation and other problems.

their lives were all about proving they were the best; the hardest workers

Athletes, on the other hand, are well aware of the importance of sleep. They are very active and so mostly sleep well anyway. Many are also in the habit of having naps to recover from rigorous training regimes. Sleep usually isn't a problem, despite the physical stresses they put themselves under.

RUNNING ON ADRENALINE

With some of the execs, Linia saw it was very different. Sleep was not a priority for them and, in fact, some boasted of how they could get by on very few hours of sleep. They considered rest a waste of their time, but although they were managing to function, sleep deprivation meant they were running on adrenaline, which isn't healthy. They had to make big decisions every day, but they were really not at their best because of lack of sleep. People think they can work long into the night and still cope with life, but unfortunately sleep really is something we cannot do without. It is central to our health.

they had to make big decisions every day, but they were really not at their best because of lack of sleep

Linia realized that she needed to take a holistic view of her patients' health and look at sleep as a pillar of wellbeing. It became clear to her that if people aren't getting enough sleep, the rest of their health strategies aren't going to succeed and her nutritional advice isn't going to work. The study of sleep became a priority for her and a key part of her work.

Sleep is just as important as eating well and taking exercise but it is all too often overlooked. We really do need to give sleep more attention, but the life we're living means that we skimp on our sleep because we think we can. In truth, it is the last thing we should be skimping on. We all know that life can feel like you're hitched to a high-speed train but when there just seems to be too much to do and you can't cope, it should be a cue to sleep more.

What helps me feel more grounded is keeping my wellbeing pillars balanced. And getting those pillars right means a greater resilience to stress – all too present in our lives! This is why some people can cope with more pressure than others and problems seem to wash off them more easily.

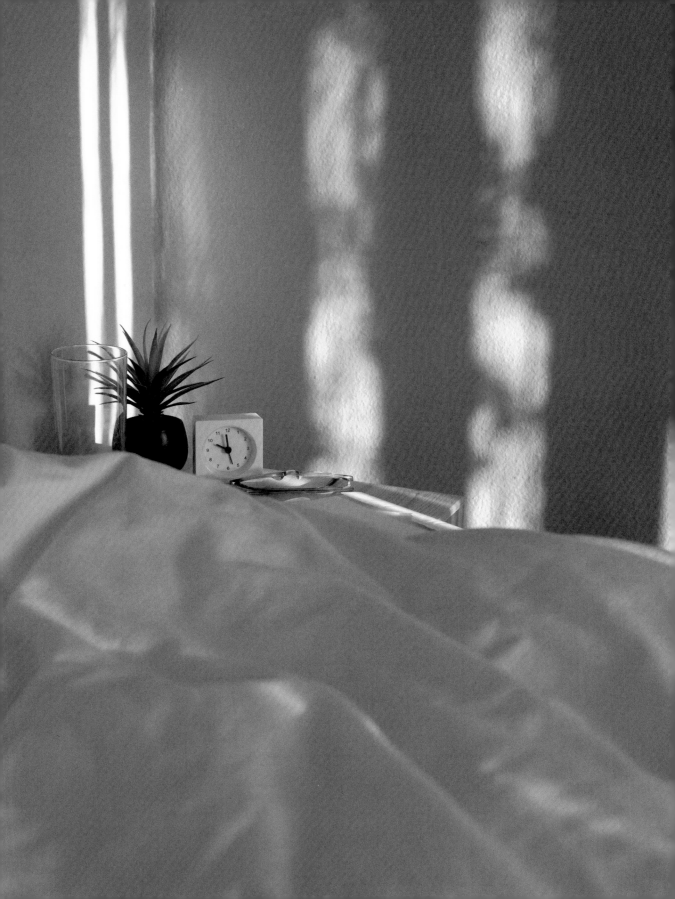

why we sleep

Sleep is not a luxury – it is essential and nearly all animals do it, but why? The reason is that the body must have sleep in order to restore itself. Sleep affects every part of the body. It allows the cells to repair and regrow through processes such as tissue growth, hormone release and protein synthesis. Without sleep, these vital processes can't happen.

Sleep helps our brain function too. When we sleep, the brain's waste-clearance system (known as the glymphatic system) clears out waste that has built up throughout the day. This allows the brain to work well when we wake up.

sleep is so important for problem-solving

Sleep also contributes to memory function converting short-term memories into long-term memories, as well as by erasing information we don't need. This might otherwise clutter up the nervous system, which is why sleep is so important for memory and problem-solving.

The science shows that when people don't sleep, the effect on the amygdala – the area of the brain involved in emotion – makes us more likely to overreact. We can get really ratty and bad-tempered because the body has had to prioritize restorative sleep over emotional processing, resulting in us being more highly strung. That saying 'He got out on the wrong side of the bed' to describe someone's bad temper has its roots in fact! For this reason, lack of sleep is linked to depression and mental health issues.

Sleep needs do change through life. A new baby may sleep for as many as 16 to 18 hours a day – although it might not feel like this to the new parents! Toddlers need about 12 hours ideally, and this gradually goes down to about 9 hours for teenagers. The National Sleep Foundation guidelines advise that healthy adults need between 7 and 9 hours of sleep per night. People over 65 should also get 7 to 8 hours per night.

TOO LITTLE SLEEP CAN MAKE YOU ILL

Research shows that after just two nights of poor sleep, your body suffers and starts releasing stress hormones. And when you're feeling stressed and you haven't slept, what do you crave in the morning? Sugar or refined carbs! You want a doughnut, not brown rice – something that pushes blood sugar levels up quickly. Lack of sleep is associated with negative health impacts like weight gain because sleep deprivation increases your appetite and makes you want more calories, particularly those from sugar and other refined carbohydrates. That croissant or bowl of cereal might raise your blood sugar so you feel better, but the relief is only temporary and the sugar-rush roller coaster begins.

lack of sleep is associated with weight gain

OWL OR LARK?

Some people love the mornings and wake up bright and cheery, but then can't string two words together after 10 p.m. Others are slow to get going in the morning but can happily work on into the small hours. Society tends to praise the early risers, the larks, but sees the night owls as lazy. Much of life is organized on the side of the larks – for example, schools start early, which just doesn't suit all children, particularly in their teenage years.

recognize your sleep habits and make the most of them

Recognize your sleep habits and make the most of them. If you naturally wake up early, you're likely to work best in the morning and fall asleep easily by 10 p.m. If you tend to wake up later, you're likely to work best in the afternoon and be able to stay up later in the evening. If possible, try to schedule your life around this to help you wake up feeling refreshed.

effects of sleep deprivation

- Studies have shown that people who sleep only 5 hours a night are four times more likely to develop a cold than those who sleep for 7 hours. Sleep supports a healthy immune system.

- Lack of sleep is thought to activate inflammatory signalling pathways in the body. Seeing these in blood tests first alerted Linia to the problems of sleeplessness in her city worker patients. Diabetes, cancer and cardiovascular disease are all linked at some level to inflammation, so too little sleep increases your risk of developing these diseases. Studies show that the shorter the sleep, the shorter your lifespan.

- Sleep has an impact on your gut health – linking it to one of the other foundations of wellness. The 'happy hormone', serotonin, is one of the building blocks for melatonin, the hormone that encourages sleep. As much as 95 per cent of our serotonin is produced in the gut and scientists believe that our gut and our sleep cycles are strongly linked. Lack of sleep is a stress on the body that affects your gut, but an imbalance of good and bad bacteria in the gut affects your ability to sleep. It goes both ways.

- Poor sleep means the skin ages faster. It doesn't recover so well from stresses like sun damage and dehydration because the regeneration isn't happening. We also get black bags under the eyes, which makes us look tired and haggard. There's nothing worse than people saying, 'You look tired.' I know that if I don't sleep well, I look 5 or even 10 years older the next day! And it's true – beauty sleep really is a thing. Linia explained to me that when we sleep well, the epidermis, the layer under the skin, gets regenerated. Sleep increases blood flow to our organs, particularly the skin, and this rebuilds collagen, which then plumps up the skin and reduces the damage done by sun exposure. This means we have fewer wrinkles and age spots. When you've slept well, you have a glow about you. Your skin thanks you and it shows. Yet another reason to get to bed early!

- Oversleeping, or consistently sleeping for more than 9 hours a night, can also have negative effects on your overall health. People who sleep too much have a decreased immune function and are likely to be overweight. They also have higher levels of inflammation in the body, which is why oversleeping increases your risk of chronic illness, such as diabetes and heart disease.

Shift work

Shift work is hugely disruptive to sleep cycles. If you work at night you're going against the body's normal circadian pattern. There is lots of research on how shift workers are at greater risk of being overweight and suffering from diabetes or heart disease because they build up a massive sleep debt over time. This has an impact both physically and mentally.

Experts are not yet sure whether the weight problems are just due to sleep deprivation or because of the foods people tend to eat around shift work – the desire for refined carbs. It does help to try to keep to as much of a regular routine as possible, even on days off, but it's not always easy. Shift workers often come home and go to bed but then only sleep until lunchtime because of noise in the house and other distractions.

Linia's advice is that little things, like wearing a sleep mask, can help. Or when you come off your shift in the morning, put on some dark glasses as a way of deactivating that daytime clock. Then, before going to work the next night, switch on lights to make your environment as bright as possible, so your internal clock says, 'Hey, get going.'

New mums

One of the most difficult times for sleep is when you have a new baby. I went back on *Strictly* 6 weeks after giving birth. I got by on adrenaline, but it was tough. Like every mother, I remember that total exhaustion that comes with getting up for night feeds and nappy changes. I don't know how I coped with those disrupted nights but, of course, I stayed in love with my baby.

What I didn't know at the time is that the body has a way to cope with this period of sleep deprivation and prepare you for it. New mothers produce a hormone called oxytocin, which gives us such a high when we look at our beloved baby. So, despite the lack of sleep and the tiredness, we are still able to love and care for the new arrival and physiologically get through this time.

what's happening
when you're asleep

As we sleep, the body goes through various cycles, which repeat a number of times during the night and vary in length between 70 and 90 minutes. There are two major stages of sleep: REM, or rapid eye movement sleep, and non-REM. As the name suggests, during the non-REM stage there is an absence of eye movement. REM is a lighter sleep and there is movement of the eyes under the eyelids. Linia explained to me what is happening during those hours of blissful unawareness.

THE SLEEP CYCLE

Stages one and two

When we first fall asleep, we enter an initial non-REM stage, which lasts only about 7 minutes. We are in light sleep and our brain waves, heart rate and eye movements slow down. If disturbed, we awaken easily. Then we go into a second non-REM stage, which is also a light sleep. So, if we take a short nap of 10 to 20 minutes in the afternoon, we obviously only go through these first two stages. The body cools down, muscles relax and our brain waves spike and slow down. Have you ever had the feeling of suddenly jerking awake? That might happen if you wake from a nap just as you enter stage three.

Stage three

In a normal sleep cycle, stage three is still non-REM and is restorative. Brain waves become even slower and your muscles relax. It is harder to wake you. This is when your body replenishes energy and repairs cells and is the stage the body prioritizes. At times when you're not getting enough sleep, it tries to go into this stage almost right away because it knows this is what you need.

Stage four

This comes about 90 minutes after we first fall asleep. Your eyes start moving from side to side under your closed eyelids and it is during this REM stage that most dreaming occurs. Your brain waves start to speed up and you might wake up briefly. In healthy sleep, you turn over and go back to sleep and the whole cycle starts again. But if you're stressed, you might keep waking up at two, three or four o'clock. What is happening is that something gets stuck as the brain is doing the emotional processing that happens in REM sleep. Somehow, the processing doesn't happen; you wake up and thoughts spiral out of control. So, if you find yourself waking in the early morning it is during that REM stage. It reveals that perhaps you have many worries or are anxious about something happening the next day.

Dreaming

Dreaming is a whole other subject and there are many different theories. It could be a way of doing a little mental therapy – clearing out what we want to remember and don't want to remember. Or perhaps it is a way of being creative or processing emotions. We may spend as much as 2 hours a night dreaming but may not remember our dreams.

Our sleep rhythm

Our body works on a circadian, which is a roughly 24-hour, rhythm and we're programmed to sleep at night and wake in the morning. Towards the evening, a hormone called melatonin, which triggers the need for sleep, increases as the light dims. That hormone release continues into the night, then decreases towards morning to prepare us for waking.

Light is a powerful factor in the whole sleep/wake cycle. My own sleep is really affected by light. I find I sleep so much better in a properly darkened room and I am easily awoken by early morning light. In the summer months, I keep an eye mask by the bed and reach for it, half-awake, as soon as I'm disturbed by those first rays of sun breaking through the blinds.

Research has shown that exposure to daylight or bright light in the morning improves sleep quality. And in the people taking part in the study, exposure to light in the morning reduced the time it took them to get to sleep by an amazing 83 per cent. Equally, dim light in the evening is important for increasing the production of melatonin to signal sleep. There is also a mechanism in the body that reminds us of the need to sleep and helps us sleep longer if we are sleep deprived.

For me, that old adage that an hour before midnight is worth two after midnight is pretty much true. It's not always possible, but I certainly feel the benefit if I go to bed early. Sleeping from roughly ten o'clock at night to six in the morning works well with our circadian rhythm. About eleven until seven is also good but really, the earlier we get on that sleep wave the better.

an hour before midnight is worth two after midnight

Of course, modern life, commuting and the feeling that we need to be in constant touch make it harder to keep to reasonable hours and get to bed well before midnight. However, think about how you can improve what you're doing in baby steps. If you find yourself turning in late every night, aim for an early night once a week, then maybe twice a week, and see how that makes you feel. It's all about small wins that are achievable. Perfection is not sustainable so just try reframing and think about making things better. Also, reframe the way you look at sleep. It is self-care, not a luxury or an indulgence.

JET LAG

Jet lag is a physical change of our circadian rhythm caused by taking ourselves to a different time zone. If it is just for a couple of days, it can be better to stay with your home rhythm to avoid messing it up too much. Otherwise, the key thing is to adapt to that new time pattern as soon as possible. You can even start before you leave by adjusting your daily routine slightly – eating a bit later or earlier, for example, depending on where you're going. When you arrive, if it's daytime, keep yourself awake until a reasonable bedtime in your new time zone. Focus on your usual bedtime routine and don't eat a heavy meal or too much sugar. Relax and try a breathing exercise or mindfulness to help you settle.

NAPS

Some people I know can curl up on a sofa and drop off anywhere, but I've never been able to do that. Linia assured me that naps are an individual thing. Either you are a napper or you're not. A short sleep in the day can be great and really refresh you. But it is all about when you have your nap and for how long. If you take a 10- to 20-minute nap, you go into the first two stages of sleep – the light sleep – and you will wake feeling restored and the better for the rest. But if you sleep for too long and are then woken up, you'll feel groggy because you've gone into deep sleep and not completed the cycle.

If you want a nap, keep it short and in the early afternoon – before three o'clock. Even if you don't actually sleep, it can help just to lie down and rest. However, if you are seriously sleep deprived, for example if you are a new mum with a baby, take the chance for a long nap that allows the full 90-minute sleep cycle and that will help.

Regular nappers don't seem to find that it affects their night-time sleep – think of those people in countries such as Spain and Italy where there is the siesta tradition. But if you just try to nap at the weekend it might not work as well, as it can disrupt your circadian rhythm and hence your sleep pattern.

sleep problems

Do you remember that Sunday-night feeling you used to have as a child when you hadn't done your homework? Still, on a Sunday night, I often find I don't sleep well because I start thinking about my to-do list for the week. For me, it's usually school- and work-related stuff that keeps me awake. I'll suddenly remember that I haven't packed the Tupperware and apron for my daughter's cookery lesson the next day and that's it. I'm awake all over again and torn between wanting to run downstairs and sort it before I forget or trying to get back to sleep. My mind starts racing, then I get anxious about not sleeping and how I'm going to cope if I don't get back to sleep. I know that many, many people experience the same thing.

don't look at your phone!

JOURNAL IT

'Before going to bed, write a list of what is in your control and what is out of your control,' says Linia. For example, organizing the children's activities is within your control, but world peace isn't! There's no point worrying about things you can't do anything about. Sometimes having that mental picture of your list can be very helpful in getting those thoughts out of the way, so make journalling – writing down a list – part of your bedtime routine.

I CAN'T SLEEP!

There are times when I've gone off to sleep fine but then wake up fretting about something I haven't done or something I have to do.

Then I lie there unable to get back to sleep. The longer it goes on, the worse it gets and I find myself thinking, 'The night is slipping away. I haven't got much longer to get some sleep and I have so much to do tomorrow.' Do I get up or just lie there and rest? It's hard to know what's best.

If you've settled in bed, turned out the lights, and then still find yourself lying awake after 25 minutes or so, don't keep looking at the clock, which just makes things worse as you see the minutes ticking away. Get up, go to another room and do something gentle and soothing to relax you. Read, listen to some music – don't look at your phone! Once you start to feel sleepy, go back to bed. That way you don't build up an association with being in bed and being unable to sleep.

If you wake up in the small hours, worrying, try this strategy. Take a thought and then choose another thought to counter it. For example, if you have a meeting coming up that you're worried about and feel you can't handle, think to yourself: hold on, I have plenty of experience and I can deal with it. I'm amazing.

Another option is to focus on the present and your breathing. When you really think about your breathing, you're too busy counting your inhalations and exhalations to bother about anything else. Instead of lying there worrying and letting lots of thoughts clutter up your brain, just breathe. You might find that before you get to 10 breaths you're off to sleep. Have a look at the breathing exercise on page 173 of this book and give this a try.

MENOPAUSE

Sleep quality does tend to be worse during menopause. Hot flushes cause a rise in temperature, though remember that your melatonin is trying to lower your body temperature so you can fall asleep. Some tips for menopausal sleep problems are to look at maximizing hormones, whether by HRT or lifestyle changes, watching caffeine and alcohol intake even more carefully, and making sure you take exercise during the day. You might also find it helpful to sleep on natural fibres, as synthetic fibres can make you warmer.

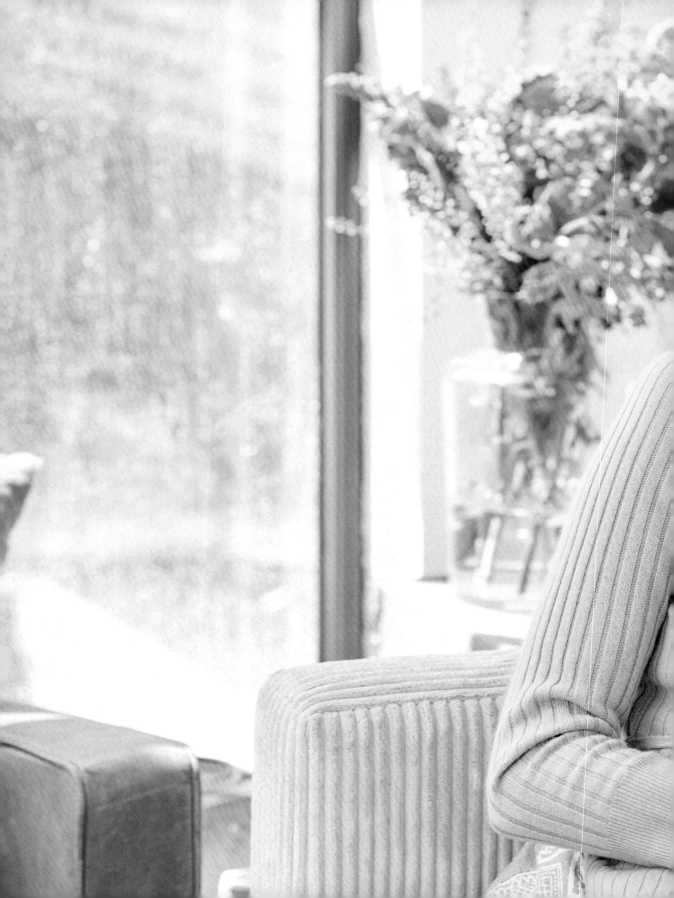

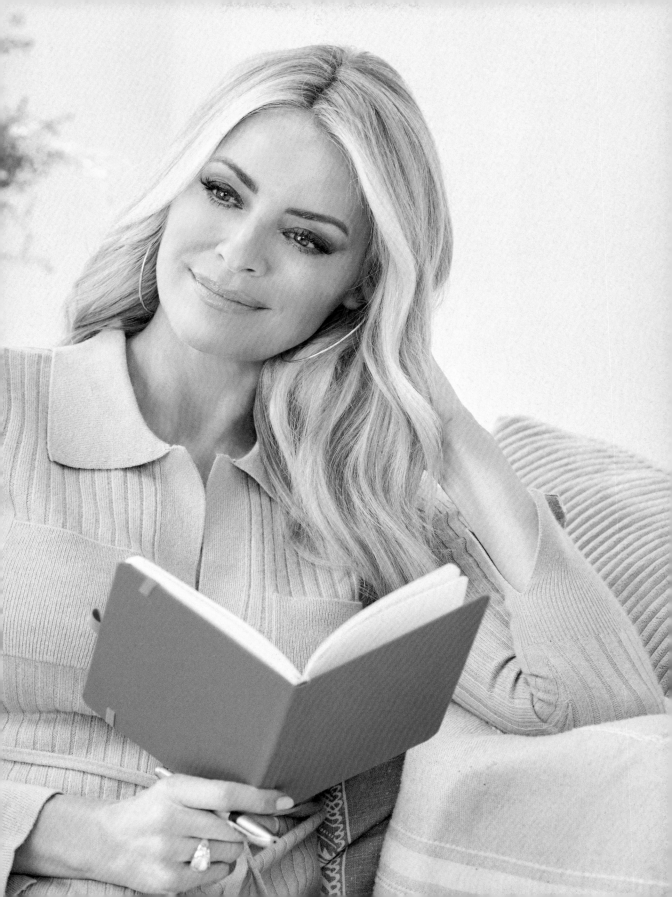

DRY MOUTH

One of my sleep problems was that I would wake up several times a night with an uncomfortably dry mouth, which really bothered me. I discovered that it was because I was breathing through my mouth all night and that was what was causing the dryness. The solution: tape up my mouth so I breathe through my nose! Sounds drastic but it's easy – just take a short strip of Micropore tape and place it vertically from just under your nose and over your lips. Don't make it too tight, just make it so it's comfortably keeping your mouth closed. Try it for 10 minutes the first night, then gradually build up the time until you get used to it. Now I wouldn't be without my bit of tape and no more waking with a dry mouth.

SLEEPING PILLS

Linia's advice is that we shouldn't rely on them. Pills do work, but you tend to wake up feeling a bit foggy and groggy the next day and sluggish. Then there's the addiction factor. Of course, there are times when people need them. For example, dementia patients often can't sleep, which makes their condition worse.

She suggests that it's better to look at all aspects of your sleep hygiene first before resorting to pills. Sleeplessness is a symptom, so look at the source of the problem. Why are you not sleeping? Is it a physical problem or psychological? What is going on in your life that might be interfering with your ability to sleep?

Natural sleep aids like magnesium, melatonin, lavender and valerian are generally considered to have fewer side effects than prescription medications, but you should still talk to your doctor before using any herbs or medications for sleep. Keep in mind, too, that any supplements are most effective when used in combination with good sleep practices and habits. They also should only be taken for the short term. If you require a little extra help to get a good night's sleep and you just want to take one supplement, then make it magnesium for a short period of time. Especially if you, like most of us, suffer from a degree of daily stress. However, as with anything, remember that more of a supplement is not necessarily better.

look at all aspects of your sleep hygiene

Before starting magnesium supplements, focus on getting the proper amount of nutrients in your diet. You can find magnesium naturally in many foods, such as dark green leafy vegetables, nuts, pulses, dairy products, soy foods and wholegrains.

SNORING

Snoring happens when the air flows through your throat as you breathe in your sleep. This causes the relaxed tissues in your throat to vibrate, which leads to snoring.

Snoring may disrupt your sleep and that of your partner. Even if it's not bothering you too much, chronic snoring is not a symptom to ignore. Speak to your doctor about it, as it may be linked to health conditions like sleep apnoea or being overweight.

Changes you can make to help with snoring:

+ Sleeping on your side. This allows the air to flow easily through your airways and your throat.

+ Raise the head of your bed. Elevating the head of your bed by a few inches may help to keep your airways more open and therefore help with snoring.

+ Limit or avoid alcohol before bed. Alcohol can relax your throat muscles, causing snoring.

+ Maintain a moderate weight. If you are overweight, weight loss will help reduce the amount of tissue in the throat. Excess tissue might be causing snoring.

+ Get enough sleep! Sleep deprivation may increase your risk of snoring. This is because sleep deprivation can cause your throat muscles to relax, making you more susceptible to airway obstruction.

INSOMNIA?

Insomnia is a sleep disorder in which you have trouble falling and/or staying asleep. The condition can be short-term (acute) or can last a long time (chronic). It may also come and go. Transient insomnia lasts for less than a week and is usually caused by recent stresses. Acute insomnia lasts from a night to a few weeks. Insomnia is chronic when it happens at least three nights a week for three months or more.

Sometimes, though, how we think we slept is very different to what is actually going on. Someone might say that they are a terrible sleeper but if you actually measure their sleep, you find they're doing OK. On the other hand, you get people who say they are sleeping well but when measured turn out to be really bad sleepers. Our own perceptions of sleep are very variable, so it's useful to think about how well you sleep.

Insomnia is linked to your mental state

Insomnia may be caused by multiple factors, including unhealthy lifestyle habits, a poor sleep environment, stress, illness and irregular sleep schedules, which disrupt the circadian rhythm, to mention but a few. It is thought that the main cause of insomnia is a state of mental or physical hyperarousal that then interferes with falling asleep or staying asleep.

Symptoms of insomnia:

+   difficulty falling asleep or staying asleep

+   disturbed sleep

+   early morning waking

+   daytime sleepiness

+   persistent worry about sleep

+   short-term effects on the ability to concentrate, forgetfulness, irritability and memory

+   depression

+   headaches

+   decreased motivation or energy

Getting a diagnosis of insomnia includes a look at your history, a physical exam and a combination of tests or procedures that are used to rule out other conditions. This might include sleep logs, home sleep apnoea tests or devices that monitor breathing, oxygen saturation and heart rate, as well as hormone tests or electrocardiograms (ECGs).

how to get a better night's sleep

Let's face it – most of us are not sleeping enough. So, how to deal with this? Initially, just try to spend enough time in bed so at least you are resting. The journey of getting yourself to sleep well can take time. Say you're usually managing less than 6 hours a night. How about aiming for 7 hours two or three nights a week? Then look at what you're doing and your sleep hygiene. Look at your bedtime routine, your eating and drinking habits and your screen use and see what you can do to make improvements. The payback? Not only will you feel better rested, but you'll be happier and healthier too.

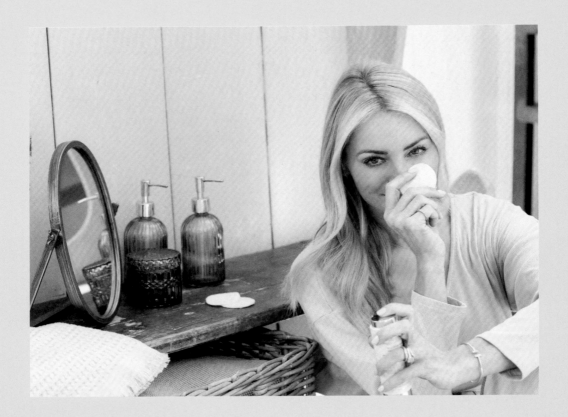

eating habits

When to eat

Eating too close to bedtime can disrupt your sleep. Ideally, have your last meal 2 hours before sleep so your body doesn't have that work of digesting. You don't want heavy food sitting in your stomach when you're trying to get to sleep. The whole idea of sleep is that your metabolism slows down because it is focusing on restoration and repair. If you are still having to digest something, your system needs energy and the metabolism doesn't slow down.

What to eat

It's also about what you eat. If you do have to eat just an hour or so before sleep, have something that is easy to digest. A big steak is hard to digest, so is definitely a no-no late in the evening. But a snack like a few olives or some fruit is easier for the body to cope with. There is a theory that carbohydrates help the production of melatonin, which makes us drowsy. Think of a pasta lunch – it makes you feel like a nap in the afternoon! This doesn't work for everyone, though, and might be to do with individual gut bacteria.

Snacking

If you find yourself snacking after supper, think about why. Are you physically hungry? If so, maybe you need to eat a bit more at your evening meal. For many of us, though, it is an emotional hunger that makes us snack, a need for comfort. We tend to use food as a reward or a consolation. Think about it – if you're physically hungry, a plate of broccoli will do the trick. But if it's emotional hunger, eating broccoli won't work and you need to have a closer look at the root cause.

Nurture your gut

Your diet can affect sleep quality. Melatonin triggers your sleep response but the precursor for it is the hormone serotonin, which is necessary for the production of melatonin. Ninety-five per cent of your serotonin is produced in your gut, so if you have a poor diet, this then impacts on your sleep. Gut bacteria thrive on a plant-based diet – that doesn't mean vegetarian or vegan, just plenty of veg and fruit. They do not thrive on refined carbs, sugar and alcohol. Research shows that if your gut isn't healthy, you are less likely to sleep well. It all connects.

avoiding stimulants

Caffeine

Tea has less caffeine than coffee, but it's best to avoid any caffeine after about three o'clock in the afternoon. A coffee in the morning is great for waking you up and getting you alert and that's why it's also good for sports performance. A marathon runner or triathlete might have some caffeine towards the end of a race because it helps them feel less tired. But it stays in the body for 6 to 8 hours, so if you have caffeine late in the day, it can impact your sleep. If you fancy a hot drink in the evening, stick with decaf coffee or herbal tea. Some people find that herbal teas such as chamomile help to relax them at bedtime and that's fine, but bear in mind that if you drink a lot of fluid in the evening, you might wake up and need the loo, which will break your sleep.

Chocolate

Remember, too, that chocolate contains caffeine, so be careful of this as well. If you're doing everything else right – avoiding screens and going to bed at a good time – you can probably cope with a couple of squares of dark chocolate, which is good for you. But if you're working at a screen and doing late nights, adding chocolate to the mix means that there are too many things going against a good night's sleep.

Alcohol

Many people say that a glass of wine or a shot of brandy makes them feel relaxed and helps them drop off to sleep. Yes, it might make you feel drowsy but unfortunately, it annihilates the quality of your sleep. You may fall asleep easily but then not sleep well. It takes quite a few hours for the alcohol to get out of your system, so a glass of wine at lunchtime might be OK in terms of bedtime, but will then wreak havoc with your afternoon!

It's all about balance though and habits. If you are drinking every night, that is clearly not good for your sleep quality. Try to plan some alcohol-free nights, particularly if you have an important day coming up and you need restorative sleep.

technology

Ditch the screens

As mentioned previously, light has a big impact on the body's production of melatonin, the hormone that helps to trigger sleep. This is why looking at your smartphone or tablet at night can be bad for sleep because that blue light from screens disrupts your melatonin production. Ideally, avoid screens for 2 hours or so before bed. Read a book instead. If you must look at screens in the evening, you can use blue filter glasses or download filters that reduce the blue light. Television screens also give out blue light, but at least we tend to sit further away from them, so the effect is reduced.

Baby steps

If the idea of being separated from your phone horrifies you, try baby steps at first. Tell yourself that you are aiming for 2 hours of phone-free time and you're starting with half an hour or an hour. Do something that calms you down instead, perhaps listening to some soothing music.

Switch off

The problem now is that we all find it so hard to switch off properly. We have the constant bombardment of social media, notifications from our phones and 24-hour news – we're on high alert all the time. I recommend switching off notifications, which really helps, and try to focus on the present – what is around you.

light

Morning

In the morning, make sure you get exposure to bright light. The evidence is that this helps to set your circadian rhythm – your body clock. Get outdoors if you can, even if it's just for a short walk or a few stretches or turn on the lights indoors.

Evening

As mentioned previously, bright light in the evening can disrupt your sleep schedule. So, if possible, dim your lights in the evening while you wind down. Take a tip from the Scandinavians and light some candles to create a warm, soothing atmosphere.

exercise

Benefits

Exercise is great for helping us reduce stress as it gets the endorphins – the happy hormones – going. Even people who don't like exercise admit it makes them feel better. We live lives that are super stressful, so it's so important to destress in a positive way and one that's good for your sleep health.

Timing

Exercise in the morning is great but it's best not to do any 2 to 3 hours before bedtime. Part of the point of exercise is to help you become alert and aware, which is not what you need in the evening. A few gentle stretches or yoga poses in the evening can help you relax, but for more vigorous exercise, make sure you're timing it right.

the bedroom

Temperature

A good temperature for your bedroom is about 18 degrees Celsius. Melatonin causes our body temperature to drop in preparation for sleep, so if the room is too hot, it takes longer for those sleep signals to work. That's why it's harder to sleep on a hot summer night. In hot countries, they keep the blinds or shutters down during the hottest part of the day to keep the room dark and cool, and only open windows later.

Black out

Keep the room as dark as possible with curtains or blinds. Some people are highly sensitive to the slightest crack of light, so wearing a sleep mask can be very helpful.

Quiet

Ideally, the room should be quiet, but that is not always within your control. If you live on a street with lots of traffic noise, for example, or you have a partner who snores, try wearing earplugs. You can also get white noise machines, which cancel out noise – some mums swear by them for helping their babies sleep.

Screen-free zone

Ban electronic devices – phones, television, laptops – from the bedroom. Keep your bedroom as a relaxing haven, away from daytime stresses.

Keep the bedroom for sex and sleep

Avoid using your bedroom for TV watching, eating or working. All these activities ruin our sleep.

bedtime routine

Preparing for bed

We're all used to setting an alarm to wake us up but how about using it to get ready for bed too? Set your alarm for 30 minutes before you want to go to bed. Otherwise you might mean to turn in at 11 p.m., but only get off the sofa just before then so you get to bed later than you planned.

Take your time

Give yourself half an hour to brush your teeth, have a shower, a warm bath, meditate or do whatever you need to do to relax. Try to make sure you're in bed with time to read a book, listen to some music or use a meditation app for a little while before you need to fall asleep.

Write it down

If you find yourself worrying about the next day and what you have to do, make a list and tell yourself it will be dealt with – tomorrow! Then put it all out of your mind.

Aids to relaxation

You can use magnesium supplements, but this nutrient can also be absorbed through the skin. A super-relaxing bath with Epsom salts before bed is a fantastic habit to get into – cheap, easy and very soothing. You could add a few drops of lavender oil for a calming aroma.

Regular bedtime

Another tip is to keep to consistent sleeping times as far as possible. People often think that because they might be sleep deprived during the week, they can catch up at the weekend by sleeping in, but that isn't the best way. It's better to keep to a regular pattern – obviously, there will be times when your social life gets in the way, and that's fine.

Waking up

The dream is to wake up naturally with the morning light, but most of us have to depend on an alarm. Setting a pleasant sound, such as music or water, might help it be less stressful or you can get devices that gradually produce light to waken you. They simulate our primeval pattern of sleeping from darkness to sunrise. It might be tempting to sleep in if you have the chance, but it's better not to as it can disrupt your sleep schedule.

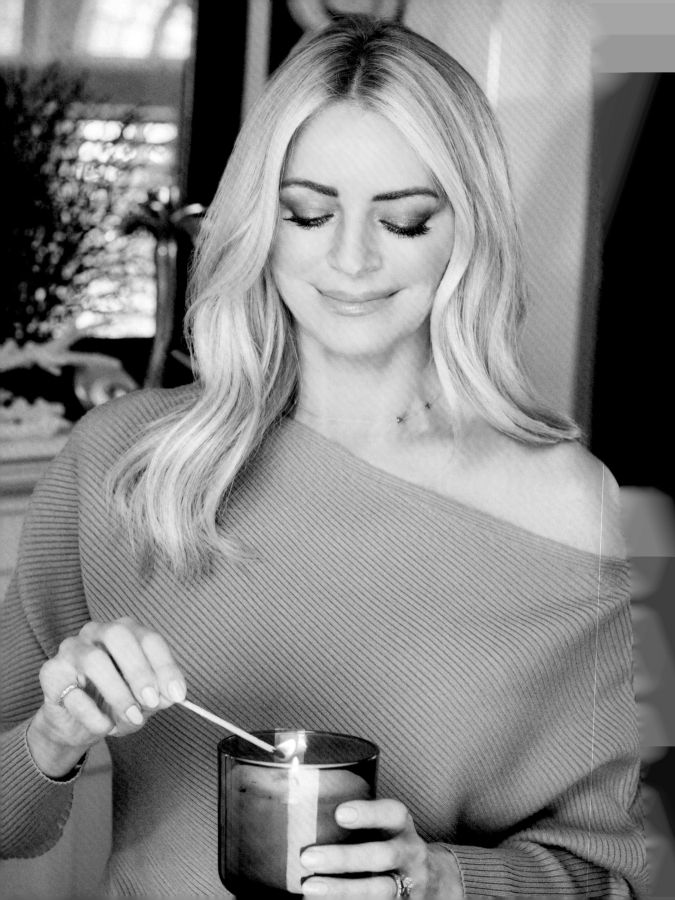

BEDTIME ROUTINE
FOR SWEET DREAMS

- **Decide on a set bedtime**. Set an alarm 30 minutes to 1 hour beforehand so you have time to prepare.

- **When it comes to nutrition, make balance your priority.** Eating a healthy balanced diet consistently has been linked with better sleep. Keeping 2 hours between your last meal and bedtime will mean that you aren't still digesting at bedtime. If you are not able to keep the 2-hour window, have a light and easy-to-digest meal based on vegetables.

- **Think about when you drink.** Be mindful of when you drink caffeine and alcohol. Limit your caffeine intake, especially in the late afternoon or evening when its stimulant effects can keep you up at night. Moderate alcohol consumption as it can throw off your sleep cycles, even it if makes you sleepy at first.

- **Switch your electronics off.** Aim for 2 hours of screen-free time ahead of your bedtime.

- **Write it down**. Thoughts, feelings, to-do lists. Get it down on paper before you sleep.

- **And chill.** Develop a bedtime ritual. Is it a bath, a book, music, breathing or meditation? What is your thing?

- **Dim the lights.** Dedicate part of your routine to turning your bedroom into a cool, dark and quiet sleep oasis.

- **Sleep well!**

a big thank you

Health and wellbeing have been foremost in my life for as long as I can remember and I'm so happy that I've been able to write this book on something that means so much to me.

I'd like to thank my publisher Kate Fox for giving me the opportunity to make this book a reality and indeed to all of the wonderful team at Transworld for their hard work and unwavering enthusiasm, including Steph Duncan, Richard Ogle, Vicky Palmer and Becky Short. Huge thanks to my brilliant team of agents at YMU – Amanda Harris, Lizzi BB, Hannah Banks and Anna Dixon – for all your support.

Huge thanks also to Jinny Johnson for your endless patience, cheerfulness, warmth (and flexibility!) when working on the book with me; and to Catherine Phipps for your help perfecting my family recipes and beyond. I also feel so fortunate to have worked with a number of wonderful experts who've shared their knowledge and experience and I'm so grateful to them for their time. A big thank you to Linia Patel (nutritionist and sleep expert), Rebecca Dennis (breathwork coach) and Sam Shaw (personal trainer).

Thank you to Georgie Hewitt who designed this beautiful book that I'm so proud of, Andrew Burton who photographed the food, and my favourite lensman of all time, David Venni, who took the photographs of me.

Last but not least, a big thank you to my gorgeous family – Vernon, Phoebe and Amber – for patiently testing recipes, listening to my ideas and generally putting up with me while I've been working on the book. Love you all.

Tess

contributors

EAT & SLEEP

Linia Patel PhD   Linia Patel is a leading dietitian and sports nutritionist. Having worked extensively in high-performance sport, she is all about helping people thrive from the inside out. She is particularly passionate about women's health and spends her clinical time working with women helping them to better understand the powerful connection between how their body works and how to achieve optimal health. Linia doesn't take a one-size-fits-all approach but sees everyone as an individual, helping them achieve their goals through a variety of methods centred around one that suits them the best. 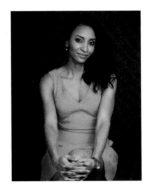 She loves science and her passion is translating nutritional science into easy-to-digest and practical advice.

Linia runs her own nutrition and dietetic consultancy, Linia Patel Nutrition, www.linianutrition.com, offering one-to-one consultations and corporate services. As a spokesperson for the British Dietetic Association she is regularly quoted in the national consumer and professional press. Linia's strong science background and vast knowledge enables her to quickly respond to breaking news stories, providing accurate background information and context. Her unique skill is translating scientific nutrition principles into simply talking about food. Outside of work Linia is a foodie and a wannabe triathlete.

MOVE

Sam Shaw   Sam Shaw is the go-to personal trainer for CEOs, celebrities and actors preparing for their next on-screen roles. He is the founder of the personal training private gym, Lemon Studios, www.lemonpt.com. His coaching ethos incorporates a multi-faceted

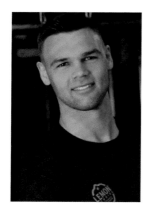

fitness and nutrition programme, specializing in physical transformation and rehabilitation.

Underpinning the Lemon Studios ideology is the simple philosophy of helping individuals achieve their personal goals through a holistic support system. His approach helps people achieve an equilibrium within physical, mental and social wellbeing, enabling them to maintain a lean, strong body and sustain a more balanced lifestyle.

Sam has been transforming lives for over a decade. His pathway to becoming a Qualified Specialist Personal Trainer resulted from his own journey overcoming obesity and its associated issues into becoming an inspiring, transformative coach.

Sam's approach is designed with the simple goal of helping people achieve the healthiest and happiest version of themselves.

BREATHE

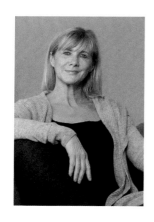

Rebecca Dennis   Rebecca Dennis, international author, breath coach and workshop leader is the founder of www.breathingtree.co.uk.

Based in London and working globally as a breath coach facilitating workshops, events and retreats alongside her public speaking, she fervently believes that conscious breathwork is the ultimate key to our wellbeing, health and inner peace.

Rebecca has been practising holistic and alternative therapies for over 20 years and has trained with many masters and influential teachers of breathwork, bodywork and healing modalities. On her journey with holistic practices, she also has trained in coaching, anatomy and physiology, Swedish and deep tissue massage, acupressure, reiki and shamanic healing traditions from indigenous tribes and elders.

Rebecca is continually inspired by the simple power of our breath and how it can change lives, including her own. She is on a mission to teach as many people as possible to empower their lives and improve their physical and mental wellbeing with conscious breathing techniques and somatic bodywork.

index

TRANSWORLD PUBLISHERS
Penguin Random House, One Embassy Gardens, 8 Viaduct Gardens,
London SW11 7BW
www.penguin.co.uk

Transworld is part of the Penguin Random House group of companies
whose addresses can be found at **global.penguinrandomhouse.com**

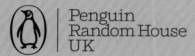

First published in Great Britain in 2023 by Bantam an imprint of
Transworld Publishers

A CIP catalogue record for this book is available from the British Library.

ISBN 9781787636422

Typeset in Cera Pro/9.5 pt
by Georgie Hewitt www.igotapapercut-studio.com
Printed in Germany

The authorized representative in the EEA is Penguin Random House
Ireland, Morrison Chambers, 32 Nassau Street, Dublin D02 YH68.

Penguin Random House is committed to a sustainable future for our
business, our readers and our planet. This book is made from Forest
Stewardship Council® certified paper.

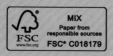